STUDY GUIDE TO

Child and Adolescent
PSYCHIATRY

A Companion to
Dulcan's Textbook of Child and Adolescent Psychiatry,
Third Edition

STUDY GUIDE TO

Child and Adolescent
PSYCHIATRY

A Companion to
Dulcan's Textbook of Child and Adolescent Psychiatry,
Third Edition

Edited by

Tapan Parikh, M.D., M.P.H.
Mina K. Dulcan, M.D.

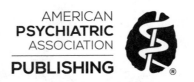

AMERICAN
PSYCHIATRIC
ASSOCIATION
PUBLISHING

Copyright © 2023 American Psychiatric Association Publishing

ALL RIGHTS RESERVED

First Edition

Manufactured in the United States of America on acid-free paper
27 26 25 24 23   5 4 3 2 1

American Psychiatric Association Publishing
800 Maine Avenue SW
Suite 900
Washington, DC 20024-2812
www.appi.org

Library of Congress Cataloging-in-Publication Data
A CIP record is available from the Library of Congress.
ISBN 9781615374915 (paperback), 9781615374922 (ebook)

British Library Cataloguing in Publication Data
A CIP record is available from the British Library.

Contents

Contributors

Nadina Abdullayeva, M.D.
Child Psychiatrist, Youth Psychiatry, The Royal Ottawa Health Care Group, Ottawa, Ontario, Canada

Shirley Alleyne, M.B., B.S.
Director, Psychiatry Residency Training Program, Lakeland Regional Health, Lakeland, Florida

Cheryl S. Al-Mateen, M.D.
Psychiatry and Pediatrics and Medical Director, Virginia Treatment Center for Children, Children's Hospital of Richmond at VCU; Program Director, Child and Adolescent Psychiatry Fellowship, Department of Psychiatry, Virginia Commonwealth University School of Medicine, Richmond, Virginia

Miya R. Asato, M.D.
Vice-President of Training, Kennedy Krieger Institute; Project Director, Maternal and Child Health Leadership Education in Neurodevelopmental Disabilities (LEND) Program; Professor, Departments of Neurology and Pediatrics, Johns Hopkins School of Medicine, Baltimore, Maryland

Rachel Ballard, M.D., M.A.
Director of Collaborative Care and Attending Psychiatrist, Pritzker Department of Psychiatry and Behavioral Health, Ann and Robert H. Lurie Children's Hospital of Chicago; Associate Professor of Psychiatry and Pediatrics, Northwestern University Feinberg School of Medicine, Chicago, Illinois

Ewa Bieber, M.D.
Assistant Professor of Psychiatry and Behavioral Sciences, Northwestern University Feinberg School of Medicine; Pritzker Department of Psychiatry and Behavioral Health, Ann and Robert H. Lurie Children's Hospital of Chicago, Chicago, Illinois

Abdullah Bin Mahfodh, M.D.
Child and Adolescent Psychiatry Fellow, McGaw Medical Center of Northwestern University, Ann and Robert H. Lurie Children's Hospital of Chicago, Chicago, Illinois

Boris Birmaher, M.D.
Distinguished Professor of Psychiatry, University of Pittsburgh Medical Center, Pittsburgh, Pennsylvania

Moshe Bitterman, M.D.
Child and Adolescent Psychiatry Fellow, McGaw Medical Center of Northwestern University, Ann & Robert H. Lurie Children's Hospital of Chicago, Chicago, Illinois

Jeff Q. Bostic, M.D., Ed.D.
Professor of Clinical Psychiatry, MedStar Georgetown University Hospital, Washington, D.C.

David A. Brent, M.D.
Distinguished Professor of Psychiatry, Pediatrics, Epidemiology, and Clinical and Translational Science and Endowed Chair in Suicide Studies, Western Psychiatric Hospital, University of Pittsburgh Medical Center, Pittsburgh, Pennsylvania

Oscar G. Bukstein, M.D., M.P.H.
Vice Chair of Psychiatry, Boston Children's Hospital; Professor of Psychiatry, Harvard Medical School, Boston, Massachusetts

Shane Burke, M.D.
Child and Adolescent Psychiatry Fellow, McGaw Medical Center of Northwestern University, Ann and Robert H. Lurie Children's Hospital of Chicago, Chicago, Illinois

Anil Chacko, Ph.D.
Associate Professor, Department of Applied Psychology, New York University, New York, New York

Judith A. Cohen, M.D.
Professor of Psychiatry, Drexel University College of Medicine, Allegheny Health Network, Pittsburgh, Pennsylvania

Steven P. Cuffe, M.D.
Psychiatry Fellowship Program Director, Department of Psychiatry, University of Florida College of Medicine-Jacksonville, Jacksonville, Florida

Lisa M. Cullins, M.D.
Training Director, PGY4 Psychiatry Residency & Clinical Fellowship Program; Intramural Research Program Attending Physician, Emotion and Development Branch, National Institute of Mental Health, Bethesda, Maryland

Eric Daleiden, Ph.D.
Partner, PracticeWise LLC, Satellite Beach, Florida

Mary Lynn Dell, M.D., D.Min.
Medical Director, Psychiatry and Behavioral Health, Children's Hospital New Orleans; Adjunct Professor of Psychiatry and Behavioral Sciences and Adjunct Instructor of Pediatrics, Tulane University, New Orleans, Louisiana

Mina K. Dulcan, M.D.
Professor of Psychiatry and Behavioral Sciences and Pediatrics, Northwestern University Feinberg School of Medicine, Pritzker Department of Psychiatry and Behavioral Health, Ann and Robert H. Lurie Children's Hospital of Chicago, Chicago, Illinois

Melissa R. Dvorsky, Ph.D.
Assistant Professor of Pediatrics and Psychiatry and Behavioral Sciences; Director, ADHD & Learning Differences Program, Children's National Hospital and Center for Translational Research, Division of Psychology and Behavioral Health, George Washington University School of Medicine and Health Sciences, Washington, D.C.

Kamryn T. Eddy, Ph.D.
Co-director, Eating Disorders Clinical and Research Program, Massachusetts General Hospital; Associate Professor, Department of Psychiatry, Harvard Medical School, Boston, Massachusetts

Graham J. Emslie, M.D.
Charles E. and Sarah M. Seay Chair in Child Psychiatry and Professor of Psychiatry and Pediatrics, Department of Psychiatry, UT Southwestern Medical Center; Child and Adolescent Psychiatrist, Children's Health, Children's Medical Center, Dallas, Texas

Elise Fallucco, M.D.
Chief and Associate Professor, Division of Child and Adolescent Psychiatry; Training Director, Child and Adolescent Psychiatry Fellowship; and Director, Center for Collaborative Care, University of Florida College of Medicine—Jacksonville, Jacksonville, Florida

Robert L. Findling, M.D., M.B.A.
Department Chair and C. Kenneth and Diane Wright Distinguished Chair in Clinical and Translational Research, Department of Psychiatry, Virginia Commonwealth University, Richmond, Virginia

Julianna Finelli, M.D.
Assistant Professor, Tulane University School of Medicine, New Orleans, Louisiana

Mary A. Fristad, Ph.D., ABPP
Director of Academic Affairs and Research Development, Big Lots Behavioral Health Services, Nationwide Children's Hospital; Professor Emerita of Psychiatry and Behavioral Health, Psychology, and Nutrition, The Ohio State University, Columbus, Ohio

Daniel A. Geller, M.B.B.S., FRACP
Founder and Director of Research, Pediatric OCD and Tic Disorder Program, Department of Psychiatry, Massachusetts General Hospital; Professor of Psychiatry, Harvard Medical School, Boston, Massachusetts

Lisa L. Giles, M.D.
Professor of Pediatrics and Psychiatry, University of Utah School of Medicine, Salt Lake City, Utah

Mary Margaret Gleason, M.D.
Kay W. Abiouness Distinguished Professor in Pediatric Psychiatry, Eastern Virginia Medical School, Norfolk, Virginia

Tina R. Goldstein, Ph.D.
Pittsburgh Foundation Endowed Professor in Psychiatry Research and Associate Professor of Psychiatry and Psychology, Western Psychiatric Hospital, University of Pittsburgh Medical Center, Pittsburgh, Pennsylvania

Karen R. Gouze, Ph.D.
Professor of Psychiatry and Behavioral Sciences, Northwestern University Feinberg School of Medicine; Psychologist, Center for Childhood Resilience, Ann and Robert H. Lurie Children's Hospital of Chicago, Chicago, Illinois

Meredith L. Gunlicks-Stoessel, Ph.D.
Associate Professor, Department of Psychiatry and Behavioral Sciences, University of Minnesota, Minneapolis, Minnesota

John Hamilton, M.D., M.Sc.
Teaching Associate in Psychiatry, Cambridge Health Alliance, Harvard Medical School, Cambridge, Massachusetts

Courtney Heim, D.O.
Child and Adolescent Psychiatry Fellow, McGaw Medical Center of Northwestern University, Ann and Robert H. Lurie Children's Hospital of Chicago, Chicago, Illinois

Sharon A. Hoover, Ph.D.
Professor of Psychiatry, National Center for School Mental Health, University of Maryland School of Medicine, Baltimore, Maryland

Anju Hurria, M.D., M.P.H.
Associate Professor of Psychiatry and Associate Training Director of Child and Adolescent Psychiatry Fellowship Program, Department of Psychiatry and Human Behavior, UC Irvine Health, Orange, California

Martha J. Ignaszewski, M.D., FRCPC
Clinical Lead Substance Use Response and Facilitation Lead, BC Children's Hospital; Education Lead Complex Pain and Addiction Service Vancouver General Hospital; Department of Psychiatry, University of British Columbia, British Columbia, Canada

Iliyan Ivanov, M.D.
Professor of Psychiatry, Icahn School of Medicine at Mount Sinai, New York, New York

Aron Janssen, M.D.
Associate Professor of Psychiatry, Northwestern University Feinberg School of Medicine; Vice Chair of Child and Adolescent Psychiatry, Pritzker Department of Psychiatry and Behavioral Health, Ann and Robert H. Lurie Children's Hospital of Chicago, Chicago, Illinois

Jessica M. Jones, M.A.
Senior Research Scientist, Department of Psychiatry, UT Southwestern Medical Center; Research Coordinator, Children's Health, Children's Medical Center, Dallas, Texas

Paramjit T. Joshi, M.D.
Professor of Psychiatry, UC Irvine School of Medicine; Director of Child and Adolescent Psychiatry Fellowship Program, Department of Psychiatry and Human Behavior, UC Irvine Health, Orange, California

Yael Kufert, M.D.
Assistant Professor, Department of Psychiatry, Icahn School of Medicine at Mount Sinai, New York, New York

MaryBeth Lake, M.D.
Associate Professor, Department of Psychiatry & Behavioral Sciences, Northwestern University Feinberg School of Medicine, and Pritzker Department of Psychiatry and Behavioral Health, Ann & Robert H. Lurie Children's Hospital of Chicago

Esther S. Lee, M.D.
Assistant Professor of Psychiatry and Behavioral Sciences, Department of Psychiatry, Johns Hopkins University School of Medicine, Baltimore, Maryland

Kelly Walker Lowry, Ph.D.
Director of Training in Psychology, Pritzker Department of Psychiatry and Behavioral Health, Ann and Robert H. Lurie Children's Hospital of Chicago; Associate Professor of Psychiatry and Behavioral Sciences, Northwestern University Feinberg School of Medicine, Chicago, Illinois

Anthony P. Mannarino, Ph.D.
Chair, Psychiatry and Behavioral Health Institute, Allegheny Health Network; Professor of Psychiatry, Drexel University College of Medicine, Pittsburgh, Pennsylvania

John S. Markowitz, Pharm.D.
Professor, Department of Pharmacotherapy and Translational Research, University of Florida College of Pharmacy, Gainesville, Florida

Emanuel Martinez, M.D.
Child and Adolescent Psychiatry Fellow, McGaw Medical Center of Northwestern University, Ann and Robert H. Lurie Children's Hospital of Chicago, Chicago, Illinois

Wendy R. Martinez Araujo, M.D.
Child and Adolescent Psychiatry Fellow, McGaw Medical Center of Northwestern University, Ann and Robert H. Lurie Children's Hospital of Chicago, Chicago, Illinois

Nicole Mavrides, M.D.
Medical Director of Child Psychiatry, PM Pediatric Care; Associate Voluntary Professor, Department of Psychiatry and Behavioral Sciences, University of Miami Miller School of Medicine, Miami, Florida

Jack McClellan, M.D.
Professor, University of Washington Department of Psychiatry and Behavioral Sciences, Seattle, Washington

Laura Mufson, Ph.D.
Viola W. Bernard Professor of Medical Child Psychology (in Psychiatry), Columbia University, Vagelos College of Physicians and Surgeons; Research Scientist, New York State Psychiatric Institute, New York, New York

Neha Navsaria, Ph.D.
Associate Professor of Psychiatry (Child), Department of Psychiatry (Child), Washington University School of Medicine, St. Louis, Missouri

Jeffrey H. Newcorn, M.D.
Professor of Psychiatry and Pediatrics, Icahn School of Medicine at Mount Sinai, New York, New York

Tapan Parikh, M.D., M.P.H.
Assistant Professor, Department of Psychiatry & Behavioral Sciences, Northwestern University Feinberg School of Medicine; Medical Director, Acute Care Services, Pritzker Department of Psychiatry and Behavioral Health, Ann & Robert H. Lurie Children's Hospital of Chicago, Chicago, Illinois

Tara S. Peris, Ph.D.
Professor and Vice Chair for Research; Associate Director, Division of Child and Adolescent Psychiatry; Program Director, ABC Children's Partial Hospitalization Program; Co-Director, UCLA Child OCD, Anxiety, & Tic Disorders Program, Jane and Terry Semel Institute for Neuroscience & Human Behavior, Los Angeles, California

Sigita Plioplys, M.D.
Head of Pediatric Neuropsychiatry Program, Pritzker Department of Psychiatry and Behavioral Health, Ann and Robert H. Lurie Children's Hospital of Chicago; Professor of Psychiatry and Behavioral Sciences, Northwestern University Feinberg School of Medicine, Chicago, Illinois

Steven R. Pliszka, M.D.
Dielmann Distinguished Professor and Chair, Department of Psychiatry, University of Texas Health Science Center at San Antonio, San Antonio, Texas

Jonathan Pochyly, Ph.D.
Instructor of Psychiatry and Behavioral Sciences, Northwestern University Feinberg School of Medicine, Pritzker Department of Psychiatry and Behavioral Health, Ann and Robert H. Lurie Children's Hospital of Chicago, Chicago, Illinois

Yann B. Poncin, M.D.
Assistant Professor of Clinical Psychiatry; Medical Director, Youth Services, Vice Chair for Clinical Affairs, Yale Child Study Center, New Haven, Connecticut

Parna Prajapati, M.D., M.P.H.
Assistant Professor of Psychiatry, Virginia Treatment Center for Children, Department of Psychiatry, Virginia Commonwealth University, Richmond, Virginia

Jennifer Rahman, M.D.
Assistant Professor, Department of Psychiatry (Child), Pediatric Integrated Mental Health Program, Columbia University Medical Center, Columbia University, New York

Jennifer B. Reese, Psy.D.
Manager of Education and Training, Big Lots Behavioral Health Services, Nationwide Children's Hospital; Clinical Assistant Professor of Psychiatry and Behavioral Health, The Ohio State University, Columbus, Ohio

Erika Ryst, M.D.
Research Associate Professor and Medical Director, Nevada Center for Excellence in Disabilities, College of Education and Human Development, University of Nevada, Reno, Reno, Nevada

Julie Mary Sadhu, M.D.
Associate Professor, Department of Psychiatry and Behavioral Sciences, Northwestern University Feinberg School of Medicine; Director of Education and of Child and Adolescent Psychiatry Fellowship Program, Pritzker Department of Psychiatry and Behavioral Health, Ann and Robert H. Lurie Children's Hospital of Chicago, Chicago, Illinois

Kris Scardamalia, Ph.D., LSSP, LP
Assistant Professor of Psychiatry, National Center for School Mental Health, University of Maryland School of Medicine, Baltimore, Maryland

Linda Schmidt, M.D.
Assistant Professor, Division of Child and Adolescent Psychiatry, and Director, Oregon Psychiatric Access-Line for Kids (OPAL-K), Oregon Health and Science University, Portland, Oregon

McKenzie Schuyler, B.S.
Clinical Research Coordinator, Massachusetts General Hospital

Craig J.R. Sewall, Ph.D., LCSW
Licensed Clinical Social Worker; Postdoctoral Fellow, Western Psychiatric Hospital, University of Pittsburgh Medical Center, Pittsburgh, Pennsylvania

Khushbu Shah, M.D., M.P.H.
Assistant Professor of Psychiatry and Behavioral Sciences, Northwestern University Feinberg School of Medicine, Pritzker Department of Psychiatry and Behavioral Health, Ann and Robert H. Lurie Children's Hospital of Chicago, Chicago, Illinois

Mark A. Stein, Ph.D.
Professor of Psychiatry and Behavioral Sciences, Department of Psychiatry and Behavioral Sciences, University of Washington, Seattle, Washington

Amanda Steinberg, B.S.
Clinical Research Coordinator, ADHD and Learning Differences Program, Children's National Hospital, Center for Translational Research, Washington, D.C.

Ronald Steingard, M.D.
Executive Editor, *Journal of Child and Adolescent Psychopharmacology*, Tufts University School of Medicine, Boston, Massachusetts

Laura A. Stone, M.D.
Associate Professor of Psychiatry, Department of Psychiatry, UT Southwestern Medical Center; Child and Adolescent Psychiatrist, Children's Health, Children's Medical Center, Dallas, Texas

Jeffrey R. Strawn, M.D.
Professor of Psychiatry, Pediatrics and Clinical Pharmacology and Associate Vice Chair of Research and Director, Anxiety Disorders Research Program, Department of Psychiatry, College of Medicine, University of Cincinnati, Cincinnati, Ohio

Anna Sunshine, M.D., Ph.D.
Acting Assistant Professor, University of Washington Department of Psychiatry and Behavioral Sciences, Seattle, Washington

Christopher R. Thomas, M.D.
Robert L. Stubblefield Professor of Child and Adolescent Psychiatry, Assistant Dean for Graduate Medical Education, and Director of Child Psychiatry Fellowship Training, University of Texas Medical Branch, Galveston, Texas

Karen Toth, Ph.D.
Alumnus-Assistant Professor, Department of Psychiatry and Behavioral Science, University of Washington, Seattle, Washington Clinical Faculty, Department of Psychology, University of Washington

John T. Walkup, M.D.
Margaret C. Osterman Professor of Psychiatry and Chair, Pritzker Department of Psychiatry and Behavioral Health, Ann and Robert H. Lurie Children's Hospital of Chicago, Chicago, Illinois

Jonathon Wanta, M.D.
Child and Adolescent Psychiatry Fellow, Pritzker Department of Psychiatry and Behavioral Health, Ann and Robert H. Lurie Children's Hospital of Chicago, Chicago, Illinois

Jill Weissberg-Benchell, Ph.D.
Professor of Psychiatry and Behavioral Sciences, Northwestern University Feinberg School of Medicine, Pritzker Department of Psychiatry and Behavioral Health, Ann and Robert H. Lurie Children's Hospital of Chicago, Chicago, Illinois

Richard Wendel, Ph.D.
Associate Professor of Clinical Psychiatry and Behavioral Sciences, Northwestern University Feinberg School of Medicine; Allied Health Professional, Ann and Robert H. Lurie Children's Hospital of Chicago, Chicago, Illinois

Ashley Winch, M.S.
Graduate, Department of Clinical Psychology, University of Central Florida, Orlando, Florida

Tareq Yaqub, M.D.
Assistant Professor, Department of Psychiatry and Behavioral Sciences, Northwestern University Feinberg School of Medicine, and Pritzker Department of Psychiatry and Behavioral Health, Ann & Robert H. Lurie Children's Hospital of Chicago

Eric Youngstrom, Ph.D.
Professor of Psychology and Neuroscience and Psychiatry, University of North Carolina; Helping Give Away Psychological Science, 501c3, Chapel Hill, North Carolina

Briahna Yuodsnukis, Ph.D.
Pediatric Psychology Postdoctoral Fellow, Gender and Sex Development Program, The Potocsnak Family Division of Adolescent and Young Adult Medicine, Ann and Robert H. Lurie Children's Hospital of Chicago, Chicago, Illinois

Charles H. Zeanah, M.D.
Mary Peters Sellars-Polchow Chair of Psychiatry and Professor of Psychiatry and Pediatrics, Tulane University, New Orleans, Louisiana

Frank Zelko, Ph.D.
Director, Pediatric Neuropsychology Service, Pritzker Department of Psychiatry and Behavioral Health, Ann and Robert H. Lurie Children's Hospital of Chicago; Associate Professor of Psychiatry and Behavioral Sciences, Northwestern University Feinberg School of Medicine, Chicago, Illinois

PART I

Questions

C H A P T E R   1

Process of Assessment and Diagnosis

Julie Mary Sadhu, M.D.

1.   Which of the following is typically *not* a focus of a psychiatric evaluation of a child in the emergency department?

A. Assessment of risk of harm to self.
B. Screening for physical abuse.
C. Planning for appropriate disposition.
D. Detailed developmental history.

2.   Which of the following questions would be best for establishing rapport when beginning an outpatient assessment of a 13-year-old adolescent?

A. Why are you here today?
B. What problems do you have that I can help with?
C. How is your relationship with your parents?
D. What grade are you in?

3.   When assessing a child's level of functioning during an assessment, what are the five main realms of functioning to consider?

A. Family, peer, school, the child's inner sense of self, and the child's inner world of fantasy.
B. Hobbies, parents, siblings, friends, and pets.
C. School, parents, siblings, friends, and work.
D. School, parents, siblings, friends, and extracurricular activities.

4.	Which of the following is *not* a benefit of using standardized rating scales in assessment?

A. Comparison of the youth with age- and gender-based norms.
B. Improved diagnostic clarity.
C. Input from individuals outside the session.
D. Elimination of the need to interview the parent.

5.	What is an advantage of the family-based approach to the initial interview?

A. The adolescent feels more comfortable talking about sexual activity.
B. The parents and adolescent may have a sense of transparency about the process.
C. The interview takes longer than the traditional approach of interviewing.
D. The adolescent is more likely to divulge details about drug use.

6.	McHugh and Slavney's (1998) model for formulation, perspectives of psychiatry, identifies four types of problems common to psychiatry. Which of the following is *not* one of these four types of problems?

A. Psychiatric diseases.
B. Disorders related to dimensional or constitutional differences.
C. Behavioral problems.
D. Epigenetic factors.

Reference

McHugh PR, Slavney P: The Perspectives of Psychiatry, 2nd Edition. Baltimore, MD, Johns Hopkins University Press, 1998

C H A P T E R 2

Assessing Infants and Toddlers

Julianna Finelli, M.D.

Mary Margaret Gleason, M.D.

Charles H. Zeanah, M.D.

1.   A 3-year-and-4-month-old boy presents with his mother for assessment of dys-regulated emotions and behaviors. The main reason that the caregiving relationship is a focus of the assessment is

A. The attachment classification determines the diagnosis.
B. The quality of the caregiving relationship with his mother reflects his other caregiving relationships.
C. The quality of the caregiving relationship may buffer against environmental risks.
D. The quality of the caregiving relationship is a good snapshot of this point in time, although it does not have predictive value.

2.   A 4-year-and-2-month-old girl is referred to you for evaluation of possible ADHD. Her father is reluctant to attend the first appointment because he thinks she is too young for any diagnostic labels to be considered. You may use which of the following in your conversation with him?

A. You let him know that DSM-5 includes developmentally specific modifications for all disorders for the preschool age group.
B. You agree that using diagnostic classifications to describe preschool clinical concerns is a problem because it results in inappropriate "labeling" without clinical value.

C. You note that insurers will not pay for the care of children's mental health problems, so using a diagnosis is not necessary.

D. You state that the multiaxial DC:0–5 provides developmentally specific evidence-informed diagnostic criteria to describe clinical mental health concerns in young children and includes a crosswalk to the DSM-5 and ICD-11 systems for billing purposes.

3.   Which of the following statements is true regarding the comprehensive assessment of infants and toddlers?

A. Evaluation should begin with focused and close-ended questions regarding the chief complaint.

B. Only formal, structured observational procedures should be used to assess the parent-child relationship.

C. Multiple appointments—involving multiple informants and modes of assessment—are typically required.

D. It is important to conduct interviews and observational assessments of the caregiver and young child individually.

4.   The clinician's goal of information gathering in the infant and toddler assessment is to elicit sufficient information to develop a biopsychosocial formulation using all five axes in the DC:0–5. Which of the following is *not* an example of these five axes?

A. Clinical disorders.

B. Temperamental traits.

C. Relational context.

D. Developmental competence.

5.   A single mother brings her 48-month-old son to the clinic, complaining that he is aggressive and oppositional and has behavior problems at both school and home. The boy is silent and looks at the floor most of the time as his mother talks to the clinician. After obtaining a detailed history of the boy's symptoms, development, social situation, family, and medical history, the clinician wants to assess the boy's attachment to his mother. The most reliable information comes from which of the following?

A. Themes in the boy's play with and without his mother present.

B. The amount of protest the boy exhibits when his mother is instructed to leave the room for a brief period.

C. The degree to which he uses his mother to resolve his distress after the reunion that follows a separation when his mother leaves the room briefly.

D. The amount of warmth his mother exhibits when describing his problem behavior.

6. In order to assess emotional regulation patterns of a 5-month-old infant with night waking and persistent crying, the clinician would be wise to select which of the following?

    A. The Crowell procedure.
    B. The still-face paradigm.
    C. The Insightfulness Assessment.
    D. Naturalistic observation of parent-infant interaction during history taking.

CHAPTER 3

Assessing the Preschool-Age Child

MaryBeth Lake, M.D.

Neha Navsaria, Ph.D.

1. A comprehensive assessment of a preschool child is ideally completed on which of the following schedules?

    A. A 2-hour session, including multiple caregivers and with a brief break.
    B. Multiple sessions on different days with more than one caregiver.
    C. Multiple sessions on different days with the same primary caregiver.
    D. Multiple sessions separated by an hour on the same day with one caregiver.

2. The format of a preschool assessment based on the Washington University School of Medicine Infant/Preschool Mental Health Clinic assessment paradigm is sequenced with caregivers according to which of the following?

    A. Semistructured observation, free play, complete history, review of observations/findings with formulation, differential diagnoses, and treatment plan.
    B. Free play, semistructured observation, complete history, review of observations/findings with formulation, differential diagnoses, and treatment plan.
    C. Complete history, free play, semistructured observation, review of observations/findings with formulation, differential diagnoses, and treatment plan.
    D. Free play, complete history, semistructured observation, review of observations/findings with formulation, differential diagnoses, and treatment plan.

3.	Functional play using objects in ways that demonstrate understanding and exploration of use and function typically occurs at what age?

  A. 6–12 months.
  B. 12–18 months.
  C. 18–30 months.
  D. 30 months or older.

4.	The attunement quality of the caregiver-child dyad refers to which of the following?

  A. Manner and extent to which limits are enforced by a caregiver.
  B. Level of attachment between caregiver and child.
  C. Extent to which the caregiver paces interactions on the basis of the child's signals.
  D. Level of physical or verbal affection expressed toward the child.

5.	Which of the following is the most appropriate cultural interpretation of observed child play during an assessment?

  A. The way in which young children engage with toys is universal and is not influenced by limited access to toys and play opportunities.
  B. Caregivers in collectivistic cultures may engage in one-to-one play less often because of expectations that children are engaged by the extended family/community.
  C. Effects of race and ethnicity are more important than contexts such as poverty and trauma.
  D. Fewer instances of child-directed play signify less parental sensitivity in the parent-child relationship.

6.	Which of the following represents the typical course of preschool diagnoses of ADHD, oppositional defiant disorder, depression, and anxiety over time?

  A. ADHD persists into school age, but oppositional defiant disorder, depression, and anxiety tend to resolve.
  B. ADHD and oppositional defiant disorder persist into school age, but depression and anxiety tend to resolve.
  C. ADHD, oppositional defiant disorder, and anxiety persist into school age, but depression tends to resolve.
  D. ADHD, oppositional defiant disorder, depression, and anxiety all tend to persist into school age.

CHAPTER 4

Assessing the Elementary School–Age Child

Tareq Yaqub, M.D.

1.   Which of the following is correct regarding interviewing a school-age child?

   A. Observations made in the waiting room should not influence assessment.
   B. Children often understand why they are presenting to the appointment.
   C. It can be helpful to start with normative, nonthreatening questions.
   D. Always meet with the parent first to have a better understanding of the child's presentation.

2.   Which of the following is true regarding suicidal thinking and behavior in school-age children?

   A. The child should not be questioned about this directly because it can increase suicidal behavior.
   B. Suicidal thinking and behavior are rarely present in this age group.
   C. Surveys have found a trend toward a gradual decline in suicidal thoughts and behavior over recent years.
   D. Detailed inquiry should be made regarding past and current history of suicidal thinking and behavior, as well as nonsuicidal self-injurious behaviors.

3.   Which of the following is the stage of Erik Erikson's stages of psychosocial development that applies to school-age children?

   A. Autonomy versus shame.
   B. Industry versus inferiority.
   C. Identity versus role confusion.
   D. Trust versus mistrust.

4.   Which of the following accurately describes the social development of school-age children?

    A. They prefer to interact primarily with their parents.
    B. They are not interested in the opinions of their peers.
    C. They begin to develop the ability to take the perspective of others.
    D. They reject rules and seek out risky behaviors.

5.   Which of the following is the reason that it is often recommended to avoid asking "why" questions to school-age children?

    A. Close-ended questions are more conversational.
    B. Asking "why" has a higher likelihood of upsetting the child.
    C. Responding to "why" questions requires analytical thinking beyond the abilities of most children this age.
    D. Asking "why" is not helpful in play therapy.

CHAPTER 5

Assessing Adolescents

Shirley Alleyne, M.B., B.S.

Steven P. Cuffe, M.D.

1. Which of the following statements on adolescent psychiatric symptom reporting is correct?

    A. Parents report more accurately on internalizing symptoms.
    B. Parents and adolescents often disagree on symptom reporting.
    C. Adolescents report more accurately on externalizing symptoms.
    D. Collateral information from external sources is seldom necessary.

2. When resistance occurs in adolescent interviews, what approach should interviewers take?

    A. Move to another topic to avoid offending the adolescent.
    B. Discontinue the interview to preserve the alliance.
    C. Use interviewing techniques to address resistance.
    D. Refocus on accessing information from the parents.

3. Which of the following techniques is used to capture the family history of mental illness in adolescent interviews?

    A. Developing a three-generation family genogram.
    B. Administering mental health rating scales to family members.
    C. Conducting interviews with multiple family members.
    D. Reviewing the medical records of family members.

4.   Why is assessing family structure important to the evaluation of adolescents?

    A. It establishes the adolescent's clinical diagnosis.
    B. It helps the clinician eliminate potential diagnoses.
    C. It establishes the transactional patterns in the family.
    D. It determines the clinician's treatment interventions.

5.   Why is it important to assess the adolescent's digital media use during the initial evaluation?

    A. It is associated with certain conditions such as autism spectrum disorder.
    B. It is associated with improved cognitive functioning.
    C. It is associated with better interpersonal relationships.
    D. It is associated with worsening mental health.

CHAPTER 6

Neurological Examination, Electroencephalography, Neuroimaging, and Neuropsychological Testing

Sigita Plioplys, M.D.

Miya R. Asato, M.D.

Frank Zelko, Ph.D.

1. Testing with MRI is indicated in which of the following clinical scenarios?

   A. A 15-year-old girl who takes valproic acid for the treatment of bipolar disorder.
   B. A 10-year-old boy with learning disorders and ADHD who often "spaces out" in class.
   C. An 8-year-old boy without significant medical history who developed stereotypic eye blinking and throat clearing.
   D. A 6-year-old boy with developmental delay and stereotypic episodes of staring and chewing behaviors.

2. Which brain waves are present during only the awake state?

   A. Delta (1–3/second).
   B. Theta (4–7/second).
   C. Alpha (8–12/second).
   D. Beta (13–20/second).

3.   When there is a clinical need for neuroimaging, which of the following neuroimaging tests is the usual first choice for children and adolescents?

A. Computed tomography (CT).
B. Magnetic resonance spectroscopy (MRS).
C. Functional magnetic resonance imaging (fMRI).
D. Magnetic resonance imaging (MRI).

4.   Which of the following has the weakest indication for neuropsychological testing?

A. To establish a clinical diagnosis of ADHD.
B. To resolve a question of whether a patient has intellectual disability.
C. To evaluate the cognitive basis of functional complaints.
D. To document changes in cognitive functioning over time.

5.   Which pattern of neuropsychological test results is common to several neurological, psychiatric, and general medical disorders?

A. Disruptions of attention, processing speed, and executive skills.
B. Disruptions of expressive/receptive language skills.
C. Lateralized sensory-motor dysfunction.
D. Significant intellectual disability.

6.   Which of the following would describe the most appropriate use of neuropsychological testing?

A. A 12-year-old girl with persistent postconcussion symptoms who had previous neuropsychological testing at age 8 years.
B. A 7-year-old boy who is undergoing an individualized education program evaluation at school for a learning problem.
C. A 15-year-old girl admitted to an inpatient psychiatric unit for active hallucinations.
D. A 10-year-old boy diagnosed with epilepsy who had previous neuropsychological testing 3 months ago.

CHAPTER 7

Intellectual Disability

Parna Prajapati, M.D., M.P.H.

Cheryl S. Al-Mateen, M.D.

Karen Toth, Ph.D.

1. Which of the following would a prudent psychiatrist managing an acute exacerbation of severe irritability and behavior change in an 11-year-old nonverbal girl with severe intellectual disability do first?

   A. Administer risperidone because it is very effective.
   B. Support the caregivers in addressing their burnout.
   C. Rule out nonpsychiatric causes of her presentation.
   D. Administer her home medications because she might have missed a dose.

2. A 16-year-old boy with severe intellectual disability is brought to his pediatrician's office for a routine checkup. The physical examination during this visit reveals multiple bite marks on both of his hands and a bald patch of scalp in the occipital region. On further inquiry, the parents report that most of the day he seemed to be in a good mood. They express concerns, however, over the patient's long-standing history of self-injurious behaviors (SIBs) of biting his hands and head banging that have not responded to 3 years of treatment with Applied Behavioral Analysis (ABA). A referral to a child psychiatrist is made at the conclusion of the visit. What pharmacological agent will the psychiatrist most likely consider in addressing the patient's self-injurious behaviors?

   A. Fluoxetine.
   B. Aripiprazole.
   C. Methylphenidate.
   D. No prescription, but a wait-and-watch approach.

3.   An evidence-based assessment for establishing a diagnosis of intellectual disability must include which of the following?

   A. Standardized intelligence test scores, adaptive assessment completed by a caregiver, genetic testing, and neurological assessment.
   B. Behavioral observations, adaptive assessment completed by a caregiver, sensory-motor assessment, and assessment of SIBs.
   C. Standardized intelligence test scores, behavioral observations, adaptive assessment completed by a caregiver, thorough physical examination, and clinical interview.
   D. Genetic testing, thorough physical examination, neurological assessment, and assessment of SIBs.

4.   The following treatments are evidence-based approaches for treating children with intellectual disability except for

   A. Cognitive behavioral therapy (CBT).
   B. Behavioral therapy (e.g., ABA therapy).
   C. Social skills therapy.
   D. Pharmacological treatment as the sole intervention.

5.   Which of the following statements is true regarding treatment outcomes for patients with intellectual disability?

   A. Comorbid ADHD can significantly improve response to treatment.
   B. The developmental course and prognosis of intellectual disability remain the same regardless of the cause of the disorder.
   C. Patients with Down syndrome show slowed development after age 11 years, whereas patients with fragile X syndrome often demonstrate accelerated development after age 11 years.
   D. With appropriate treatments, some individuals gain in adaptive functioning and may no longer meet the criteria for a diagnosis of intellectual disability.

CHAPTER 8

Autism Spectrum Disorders

Jennifer Rahman, M.D.

1. Which DSM-5 severity level of classification for autism spectrum disorder would be most appropriate for a child with incomprehensible speech and significant difficulty in all functional domains?

    A. Level 1.
    B. Level 2.
    C. Level 3.
    D. Level 4.

2. Which of the following is considered a gold standard assessment tool for autism spectrum disorder that combines standardized questions in conversation with semistructured play in activities?

    A. Autism Diagnostic Interview–Revised (ADI-R; Rutter et al. 2013).
    B. Autism Diagnostic Observation Schedule, Second Edition (ADOS-2; Lord et al. 2012).
    C. Childhood Autism Rating Scale, Second Edition (CARS-2; Schopler et al. 2010).
    D. Modified Checklist for Autism in Toddlers, Revised With Follow-up (M-CHAT-R/F; Robins et al. 2014).

3. Which of the following is a cognitive theory of autism spectrum disorder that refers to the difficulty in thinking from another's perspective?

    A. Weak central coherence.
    B. Decreased long-range connectivity.
    C. Extreme male brain theory.
    D. Weak theory of mind.

4. Which of the following interventions for autism spectrum disorder involves deconstructing target skills and teaching steps in progression until mastery?

    A. Applied Behavioral Analysis (ABA).
    B. Joint Attention, Symbolic Play, Engagement, and Regulation (JASPER).
    C. Picture Exchange Communication System (PECS).
    D. Social Communication, Emotional Regulation, Transactional Support (SCERTS).

5. Which two medications are FDA approved for reducing symptoms of irritability and agitation in people with autism spectrum disorder?

    A. Fluoxetine and citalopram.
    B. Risperidone and aripiprazole.
    C. Haloperidol and fenfluramine.
    D. Atomoxetine and guanfacine.

References

Lord C, Rutter M, DiLavore PC, et al: Autism Diagnostic Observation Schedule, Second Edition (ADOS-2) Manual (Part I): Modules 1–4. Torrance, CA, Western Psychological Services, 2012

Robins DL, Casagrande K, Barton M, et al: Validation of the Modified Checklist for Autism in Toddlers, Revised With Follow-Up (M-CHAT-R/F). Pediatrics 133(1):37–45, 2014 24366990

Rutter M, Le Couteur A, Lord C: ADI-R: Autism Diagnostic Interview Revised. Los Angeles, CA, Western Psychological Services, 2013

Schopler E, Van Bourgondien M, Wellman G, et al: The Childhood Autism Rating Scale, 2nd Edition (CARS). Los Angeles, CA, Western Psychological Services, 2010

CHAPTER 9

Communication Disorders, Specific Learning Disorder, and Motor Disorder

Moshe Bitterman, M.D.

1. What is the most prevalent DSM-5 communication disorder?

   A. Childhood-onset fluency disorder (stuttering).
   B. Social pragmatic communication disorder.
   C. Specific learning disorder with impairment in reading.
   D. Speech sound disorder.

2. Which of the following is not a cause of speech sound disorder?

   A. Atypical muscle tone.
   B. Auditory processing disorders.
   C. Delayed phonological knowledge of speech sounds.
   D. Receptive language deficit.

3. Untreated language disorders increase the risk of which one of the following?

   A. ADHD.
   B. Anxiety disorders.
   C. Self-injury.
   D. Substance use.

4.   Which of the following specific learning disorders is not in DSM-5?

   A. Learning disorder with impairment in mathematics.
   B. Learning disorder with impairment in reading.
   C. Learning disorder with impairment in written expression.
   D. Nonverbal learning disorder.

5.   Which of the following aspects of a specific learning disorder with impairment in reading is not captured by the more commonly used term *dyslexia*?

   A. Problems with fluent or accurate word recognition.
   B. Problems with reading comprehension.
   C. Problems with spelling.
   D. Problems with word decoding.

6.   A 5-year-old boy has had difficulty making friends at school, often feeling that people make fun of him. Teachers say that he usually responds appropriately to instructions in class, but he has trouble explaining what is bothering him when distressed. What is the most likely diagnosis?

   A. ADHD.
   B. Childhood-onset fluency disorder (stuttering).
   C. Social (pragmatic) communication disorder (SPCD).
   D. Specific language impairment.

7.   A 10-year-old girl with ADHD is noted to have limited vocabulary, poor spelling, and avoidance of written schoolwork. What is the most likely diagnosis, in addition to ADHD?

   A. Social pragmatic communication disorder.
   B. Specific language impairment.
   C. Specific learning disorder with impairment in reading.
   D. Specific learning disorder with impairment in written expression.

CHAPTER 10

Attention-Deficit/ Hyperactivity Disorder

Steven R. Pliszka, M.D.

1.   Which response best represents the findings of large epidemiological studies regarding the prevalence of the treatment of ADHD?

   A. Nearly 20% of children in the United States are being treated with stimulants at any given time.
   B. Only about 20% of children with ADHD are being treated with medication.
   C. Less than 10% of children with ADHD have received a behavioral treatment for ADHD.
   D. Nearly one-fourth (23%) of children with ADHD have received no treatment at all.

2.   A 10-year-old child presents with a history of inattention and poor grades since first grade. An ADHD rating scale from the teacher places her in the top 95th percentile for inattention symptoms but at the 50th percentile for impulsivity/hyperactivity. The patient also reports depression nearly every day, low self-esteem due to her difficulties in school, low motivation, early morning awakening, and passive suicidal ideation with no history of suicide attempts or self-injurious behavior. This clinical picture is most consistent with which of the following?

   A. Concurrent diagnoses of ADHD and major depressive disorder (MDD).
   B. ADHD with secondary demoralization due to school failure.
   C. Primary MDD misdiagnosed as ADHD in the past.
   D. ADHD and MDD, but stimulant treatment contraindicated because of risk of inducing more suicidal ideation.

3. Which of the following statements is true regarding the genetics of ADHD?

    A. Mutations in the dopamine transporter show major gene effects and predict response to methylphenidate.
    B. Only 30% of the variance in ADHD symptoms can be attributed to genetics, and the rest is attributable to the environment.
    C. In one study, more than 300 gene variants in 12 different chromosomal locations were related to ADHD risk, indicating that ADHD is a polygenic condition.
    D. Deletions and duplications in the DNA (copy number variants) are principally responsible for the genetic risk of ADHD.

4. In neuropsychological testing, in which area are deficits most likely to be found in children with ADHD compared with control subjects?

    A. Working memory.
    B. Inhibitory control.
    C. Sustained attention.
    D. Response to reward.

5. Which statement best describes the findings of the European ENIGMA-ADHD study with regard to the cortical surface area in a person with ADHD relative to control subjects?

    A. No differences relative to control subjects were found in cortical surface area in either adults or children.
    B. Smaller cortical surface area was found in frontal, cingulate, and temporal regions, with stronger effects in the child sample.
    C. The effect size of the cortical surface area was quite large, approximately 0.6.
    D. Smaller cortical surface area relative to control subjects was greater in adults than children.

6. Which of these treatments for ADHD has *not* been shown to be efficacious in randomized controlled trials?

    A. Methylphenidate.
    B. Behavior therapy.
    C. Electroencephalographic neurofeedback.
    D. Viloxazine.

C H A P T E R   1 1

Oppositional Defiant Disorder and Conduct Disorder

Christopher R. Thomas, M.D.

1. Which of the following is the central feature of oppositional defiant disorder (ODD)?

   A. Frequent arguments.
   B. Conflict with authority.
   C. Rule breaking.
   D. Irritability.

2. Along with ADHD and mood disorders, which of the following is the most relevant comorbid diagnosis for patients with ODD?

   A. Autism spectrum disorder.
   B. Anxiety disorders.
   C. Developmental learning disorders.
   D. Intellectual disability.

3. Which of the following prevention programs has the most extensively tested proven efficacy in reducing disruptive behaviors among at-risk children?

   A. The Incredible Years.
   B. Nurse-Family Partnership.
   C. Families and Schools Together.
   D. Reconnecting Youth.

4. On the basis of longitudinal studies, what percentage of youth with a diagnosis of conduct disorder (CD) go on to have antisocial personality disorder as an adult?

    A. 20%.
    B. 30%.
    C. 40%.
    D. 50%.

5. Which of the following programs is contraindicated in the treatment of youth with conduct disorder?

    A. Parent Management Training—The Oregon Model.
    B. Multisystemic therapy.
    C. Problem-solving skills training.
    D. Scared Straight.

6. Youth with callous and unemotional traits are more likely to exhibit which of the following behaviors?

    A. Sensitivity to punishment.
    B. Isolative behaviors.
    C. Thrill seeking.
    D. Anxiety.

CHAPTER 12

Substance Use Disorders and Addictions

Martha J. Ignaszewski, M.D., FRCPC

Oscar G. Bukstein, M.D., M.P.H.

1. Dr. Smith is a second-year pediatric resident rotating through child and adolescent psychiatry. She is assessing a 13-year-old adolescent girl with a presenting complaint of "overthinking" who meets diagnostic criteria for generalized anxiety disorder. During a thorough review of systems, Dr. Smith learns that the adolescent has used alcohol socially to reduce concerns about negative evaluation by peers and on two occasions has consumed alcohol resulting in blackout and vomiting. The youth's parents are alarmed about the consequences of alcohol use and ask Dr. Smith about the frequency of alcohol use in adolescents. How should she respond?

    A. Dr. Smith should inform the youth's parents that she meets the criteria for a severe alcohol use disorder and that inpatient rehabilitation treatment is indicated.
    B. Dr. Smith should provide education that early adolescence is a period of initiation of substance use, and epidemiological data reveal that adolescents have increasing use of all substances from age 12 through adulthood. Dr. Smith should suggest that further evaluation of the frequency of use and associated negative consequences are needed to guide interventions.
    C. Dr. Smith should normalize adolescent substance use, given that experimentation with substances occurs in this age range.
    D. Dr. Smith should defer this conversation to an addiction specialist because the topic of adolescent substance use is out of her scope of practice.

2. Screening for adolescent substance use is recommended in primary care and emergency department settings and can be performed by using evidence-based screening tools for youth. These may be targeted or universal screens depending on the clinical setting, presenting complaint, and presence of associated risky behaviors. Presence of which of the following suggests that targeted screening, rather than universal screening, may be sufficient because of lack of association with higher risk status?

    A. Mental health treatment.
    B. Forensic or juvenile justice involvement.
    C. Concerns requiring the involvement of child welfare or protective service agencies.
    D. None of the above. Connection with any of the above services is sufficient to require universal screening.

3. Many adolescents who use substances have psychiatric comorbidity, including both internalizing and externalizing disorders. Which of the following is best when considering psychostimulant selection for pharmacological management of ADHD in adolescents, especially considering the potential for abuse and diversion?

    A. Dextroamphetamine.
    B. Adderall XR.
    C. Evekeo ODT.
    D. Vyvanse.

4. Which of the following is not a recommended primary goal of adolescent substance use treatment?

    A. Controlled use.
    B. Abstinence.
    C. Harm reduction.
    D. Improved psychosocial functioning.

5. Which of the following is not a first-line medication used to treat adolescent opioid use disorder?

    A. Methadone.
    B. Suboxone.
    C. Hydromorphone.
    D. Naltrexone.

CHAPTER 13

Depressive and Disruptive Mood Dysregulation Disorders

Boris Birmaher, M.D.

1. Which of the following is true regarding major depressive disorder (MDD) in youth?

   A. Its symptoms are similar to MDD in adults, but cognitive development of the child and possible difficulties expressing certain symptoms should be considered.
   B. It is not usually accompanied by comorbid disorders.
   C. It does not last as long as it does in adults.
   D. It does not run in families.

2. A 15-year-old adolescent with MDD, moderate psychosocial impairment, and family conflicts was treated with supportive and family therapy for 6 weeks with partial response. Which of the following treatments should be offered next?

   A. Continue the same psychotherapy until there is a better response.
   B. Offer a trial of an antidepressant medication with an appropriate dosage and duration of treatment.
   C. Add an omega-3 supplement.
   D. Refer the patient to a partial hospitalization program.

3.   A 16-year-old female adolescent was successfully treated for an acute episode of MDD with psychotherapy and an antidepressant. To prevent further depressive episodes, which of the following options should the clinician consider?

A. Continue psychotherapy and the same pharmacological treatment for 6–12 months at the dose that helped the patient.
B. Discontinue both psychotherapy and medication.
C. Discontinue psychotherapy and continue with medication only.
D. Continue psychotherapy but discontinue medication.

4.   According to a meta-analysis, the average response to selective serotonin reuptake inhibitors (SSRIs) is 61%, compared with 50% for placebo. Which of the following is *not* true regarding the high placebo response rate with the use of SSRIs for youth with MDD?

A. Medication dose is not usually a factor in explaining a high placebo response rate.
B. The inclusion of youth with mild depression leads to a higher placebo response rate.
C. The high placebo response rate does not correlate with the number of sites for clinical trials.
D. The presence of comorbid disorders influences the rates of response or remission.

5.   An adolescent with MDD was treated with an antidepressant, but a few days later, he became more agitated and experienced worsening of suicidal ideation. Which of the following is true regarding the worsening of this adolescent's clinical status?

A. About 10% of adolescents treated with SSRIs or serotonin-norepinephrine reuptake inhibitors (SNRIs) may develop or experience worsening of suicidal ideation.
B. Suicidal ideation and suicide attempts are commonly seen in adolescents with MDD. Thus, the suicidal ideation may have existed before the youth started the antidepressant, or it may have worsened before the antidepressant began to exert its effect.
C. It is a clear case in line with the FDA black box warning that the antidepressants increase or worsen suicidal thoughts.
D. This may be antidepressant-induced activation that indicates the presence of bipolar disorder.

6. A 12-year-old girl was treated with the appropriate dose of an antidepressant for an adequate duration but without adequate response. Which of the following is the most appropriate next step?

    A. Stop the antidepressant and start psychotherapy.
    B. Admit her to the hospital.
    C. Combine pharmacotherapy with psychotherapy, preferentially cognitive-behavioral therapy (CBT) for depression.
    D. Add a second-generation antipsychotic.

C H A P T E R   1 4

Bipolar Disorder

Shane Burke, M.D.

1. Which of the following is a required criterion in DSM-5 (American Psychiatric Association 2013) for bipolar II disorder and not for bipolar I disorder?

    A. Episodes are not attributable to the physiological effects of a substance.
    B. Presence of one current or past major depressive episode.
    C. Presence of mood-congruent psychotic features.
    D. Presence of rapid cycling.

2. DSM-5 criteria for bipolar disorder have evolved over time, and bipolar disorder has subsequently become more narrowly defined. Some children and adolescents who formerly would have been diagnosed with a broadly defined bipolar disorder have been recategorized to the diagnosis of which of the following?

    A. Major depressive disorder.
    B. Dysthymia.
    C. Disruptive mood dysregulation disorder.
    D. Oppositional defiant disorder.

3. Research studies suggest that which of the following brain structures has a significant role in bipolar disorder, particularly in the emotional dysregulation aspect of the disorder?

    A. Hippocampus.
    B. Thalamus.
    C. Amygdala.
    D. Basal ganglia.

4. Which of the following is a positive prognostic factor in bipolar disorder?

    A. Older age at first symptoms.
    B. Presence of self-injurious behavior.
    C. Comorbidity with ADHD.
    D. Lower socioeconomic status.

5. Which of the following is *not* an appropriate intervention for bipolar disorder?

    A. Dialectical behavior therapy for adolescents.
    B. Psychoeducation to the patient and family about bipolar disorder.
    C. Light therapy.
    D. Addressing the educational aspects of the disorder through an Individualized Education Program (IEP) or 504 plan.

6. A 16-year-old male adolescent is admitted to an inpatient unit because of symptoms that include 7 days of euphoric mood, impulsive behavior, racing thoughts, decreased need for sleep, and pressured speech. He has no past medical history. History is significant for one past major depressive episode. The urine drug screen is negative. Which of the following is an FDA-approved treatment for his current presentation?

    A. Aripiprazole.
    B. Lamotrigine.
    C. Lurasidone.
    D. Oxcarbazepine.

7. When considering treatment of bipolar depression in adolescents, which of the following is true?

    A. Quetiapine is effective.
    B. There is no increase in risk when using a selective serotonin reuptake inhibitor (SSRI).
    C. Olanzapine-fluoxetine combination (OFC) is effective.
    D. SSRIs are the first-line treatment.

Reference

American Psychiatric Association: Diagnostic and Statistical Manual of Mental Disorders, 5th Edition. Arlington, VA, American Psychiatric Association, 2013

C H A P T E R   1 5

Anxiety Disorders

Jeffrey R. Strawn, M.D.
Tara S. Peris, Ph.D.
John T. Walkup, M.D.

1.   A 9-year-old girl presents to a clinician for an evaluation of increasing anxiety in social situations and avoidance of friends at school. She denies any significant depressive symptoms or symptoms of ADHD. At school, she continues to do well academically but cannot participate in group activities, raise her hand to ask questions in class, or spend the night with friends and describes extreme discomfort in crowds. Her clinician is considering a provisional diagnosis of social anxiety disorder. Which of the following would increase her risk of having an anxiety disorder?

   A. Behavioral inhibition.
   B. Low levels of family accommodation.
   C. The patient's biological sex.
   D. A lack of history of early childhood adversity.

2.   A 15-year-old adolescent presents with symptoms of generalized anxiety disorder. He has been working in cognitive-behavioral therapy (CBT) with his therapist weekly for 8 weeks. Which of the following components is associated with improvement in children and adolescents with anxiety disorders who are treated with CBT?

   A. Having a female therapist.
   B. Having a gender concordant patient-therapist dyad (e.g., a male therapist with a male patient).
   C. More time spent on challenging tasks and exposures.
   D. Extensive psychoeducation.

3.	Which class of medications is associated with greater and faster improvement in anxiety symptoms in children and adolescents who have generalized, separation, and/or social anxiety disorders?

	A. α_2-Agonists.
	B. Benzodiazepines.
	C. Serotonin-norepinephrine reuptake inhibitors (SNRIs).
	D. Selective serotonin reuptake inhibitors (SSRIs).

4.	A 10-year-old boy presents with anxiety symptoms that have been increasing over the past 8 months and are not associated with any recent environmental changes or external factors. He worries about his parents, getting into car accidents, becoming ill, and making mistakes. His parents describe him as "self-conscious." He frequently apologizes and worries that he has upset teachers, classmates, and parents. He notes high levels of tension and restlessness, struggles to fall asleep, and has a sleep latency of 90 minutes. His child and adolescent psychiatrist has recommended a combination of psychotherapy and medication and begins him on sertraline 12.5 mg/day. The child and adolescent psychiatrist wishes to track his symptoms over the course of treatment. Which would be the most appropriate instrument?

	A. Hamilton Anxiety Rating Scale (HAM-A).
	B. Screen for Child Anxiety Related Emotional Disorders (SCARED).
	C. Kiddie Schedule for Affective Disorders and Schizophrenia (K-SADS).
	D. Anxiety Disorders Interview Schedule (ADIS).

5.	When used earlier in adolescence, which of the following substances or medications has been associated with panic-related symptoms later in adolescence?

	A. Nicotine.
	B. Alcohol.
	C. SSRIs.
	D. Methylphenidate.

6.	In addition to SSRIs, which of the following medications has had positive studies in pediatric patients with anxiety disorders?

	A. Guanfacine extended release.
	B. Selegeline (transdermal).
	C. Vortioxetine.
	D. Alprazolam.

7.	Which of the following DSM-5 (American Psychiatric Association 2013) anxiety disorders is typically the first to emerge in children and adolescents?

	A. Generalized anxiety disorder.
	B. Social anxiety disorder.
	C. Panic disorder.
	D. Specific phobia.

Reference

American Psychiatric Association: Diagnostic and Statistical Manual of Mental Disorders, 5th Edition. Arlington, VA, American Psychiatric Association, 2013

CHAPTER 16

Posttraumatic Stress Disorder and Persistent Complex Bereavement Disorder

Judith A. Cohen, M.D.

Anthony P. Mannarino, Ph.D.

1. Which of the following is true with regard to epidemiology, risk factors, and co-morbidity related to PTSD in children and adolescents?

    A. Greater trauma exposure and a previous history of anxiety disorder are risk factors for developing PTSD.
    B. PTSD is equally common in female and male children and adolescents, and genotype does not contribute to the risk of developing PTSD.
    C. Media viewing does not contribute to increased risk for developing PTSD postdisaster.
    D. Psychiatric comorbidity occurs in less than 30% of cases in the presence of pediatric PTSD.

2. Which of the following should be included during the initial clinical evaluation of a child who may have pediatric PTSD?

    A. Assessing the child's trauma exposure and symptoms through the use of multiple informants, clinical interviews, and standardized instrument(s).
    B. Interviewing only the child about their traumatic experiences and symptoms in order to preserve the child's confidentiality and trust.

C. Not asking directly about trauma exposure or symptoms because the clinician has not yet developed a trusting relationship with the child.

D. Requiring the child to describe all of the details of their traumatic experience(s) in order to master avoidance.

3. For children diagnosed with PTSD who do not have immediate safety concerns or apparent comorbidity, what is the initial treatment of choice?

A. An evidence-based trauma-focused psychotherapy.

B. A selective serotonin reuptake inhibitor (SSRI).

C. Combined treatment with an evidence-based trauma-focused psychotherapy plus an SSRI.

D. Tailoring pharmacotherapy to address the child's most prominent PTSD symptoms.

4. During an initial evaluation, a 12-year-old boy endorses, and his mother confirms, that he was exposed to domestic violence perpetrated on his mother when he was 6–8 years old. He has significant current behavioral dysregulation. Which of the following would be a reason *not* to refer the patient to trauma-focused cognitive-behavioral therapy (TF-CBT)?

A. The family's desire to receive behavioral- rather than trauma-focused treatment first.

B. Presence of significant depressive, anxiety, externalizing behavior, and PTSD symptoms.

C. A history of early complex interpersonal trauma, significant behavioral problems, and PTSD symptoms.

D. The mother's statement that she may not be able to participate regularly in her son's treatment because of her work schedule.

5. According to preliminary evidence, which of the following appears to be an effective approach for children with maladaptive grief responses such as persistent complex bereavement disorder?

A. Providing integrated trauma- and grief-focused interventions.

B. Providing support groups for surviving parents with no child intervention.

C. Providing pharmacotherapy for depressive symptoms of persistent complex bereavement disorder.

D. Providing rebirthing or holding therapy.

6. The cognitive-behavioral intervention for trauma in schools (CBITS) has similar components as in TF-CBT. Which of the following is correct when CBITS is compared with TF-CBT?

A. CBITS is delivered as group therapy.

B. CBITS ensures parental presence.

C. Trauma narrative is an important component of TF-CBT but not CBITS.
D. The acronym PRACTICE summarizes the core components of CBITS: psycho-education and parenting skills, relaxation, affective modulation, cognitive processing, trauma narration and processing, in vivo mastery of trauma reminders, conjoint child-parent sessions, and enhancing safety.

CHAPTER 17

Obsessive-Compulsive Disorder

Daniel A. Geller, M.B.B.S., FRACP

McKenzie Schuyler, B.S.

1. Although DSM-5 (American Psychiatric Association 2013) uses the same diagnostic criteria for OCD affecting children and adolescents as for adults, pediatric-onset OCD is distinct in several important ways, including which of the following?

    A. A distinct pattern of OCD symptoms that follow developmental themes and distinct psychiatric comorbidity.
    B. Lower familial occurrence in first-degree relatives.
    C. An adolescent peak of age at onset.
    D. A poorer prognosis than for adult-onset OCD.

2. Involvement of family members in OCD behaviors in youth with OCD, known as *family accommodation*, is common. Which of the following is true regarding addressing family accommodation?

    A. It requires disengagement of accommodating family members in order to provide effective cognitive-behavioral therapy (CBT).
    B. It will enhance avoidance behaviors that are needed to decrease rituals.
    C. It can be quantitatively assessed using a family accommodation scale.
    D. It has little impact on treatment outcome.

This chapter is dedicated to the memory of Henrietta Leonard, M.D., esteemed clinician, researcher, teacher, mentor, and colleague.

3. Clinical assessment and diagnosis of pediatric OCD are best made in which of the following ways?

   A. Administering the Children's Yale-Brown Obsessive-Compulsive Scale (CY-BOCS; Scahill et al. 1997) to the affected youth.
   B. Using simple age-appropriate probes followed by a more detailed inquiry regarding time occupied by symptoms and the degree of impairment and distress experienced.
   C. After excluding potential differential diagnoses such as autism spectrum disorder and ADHD.
   D. After evaluating for pediatric autoimmune neuropsychiatric disorder associated with streptococcal infections (PANDAS) by clinical inquiry, anti-strep antibody titers, and throat swab where indicated because PANDAS may mimic OCD in youth.

4. Which of the following is true about evidence-based treatments for pediatric OCD?

   A. They are less effective for children with severe symptoms at baseline.
   B. They first require adequate management of comorbid illnesses.
   C. They cannot be delivered remotely using telehealth.
   D. They include CBT, pharmacotherapy with a selective serotonin reuptake inhibitor (SSRI), and combined treatment.

5. Which of the following is true regarding CBT for OCD?

   A. It should always be delivered as monotherapy before medicines are introduced.
   B. It has the highest documented effect size outcomes when delivered in a rigorous protocol-driven module.
   C. It is a form of relaxation therapy employing principles of acceptance and commitment.
   D. It can be delivered only by CBT-trained therapists.

6. Which of the following is true regarding pharmacotherapy for pediatric OCD?

   A. It has high rates of serious adverse events and is a last resort in treatment.
   B. Pharmacotherapy improves about one-third of children who receive medication.
   C. It has modest effects, with typical decreases in CY-BOCS scale scores of 6–8 points compared with placebo.
   D. It will show maximum benefits within 8 weeks.

References

American Psychiatric Association: Diagnostic and Statistical Manual of Mental Disorders, 5th Edition. Arlington, VA, American Psychiatric Association, 2013

Scahill L, Riddle MA, McSwiggin-Hardin M, et al: Children's Yale-Brown Obsessive Compulsive Scale: reliability and validity. J Am Acad Child Adolesc Psychiatry 36(6):844–852, 1997 9183141

CHAPTER 18

Early-Onset Schizophrenia

Anna Sunshine, M.D., Ph.D.

Jack McClellan, M.D.

1.   Which of the following environmental risk factors increase the risk of developing schizophrenia?

    A. Prenatal famine exposure and prenatal infection exposure.
    B. Cold and aloof parenting and prenatal famine exposure.
    C. Prenatal infection exposure and cool and aloof parenting.
    D. Living in a rural location and prenatal famine exposure.

2.   Fran is a 16-year-old with a diagnosis of early-onset schizophrenia (EOS) who is presenting to your clinic to establish care. After you review her previous records, which of the following would raise your suspicions for an alternative diagnosis?

    A. Fran does not have any relatives with a schizophrenia diagnosis.
    B. Fran had genetic testing, which revealed a low polygenic risk score for schizophrenia.
    C. Fran had an MRI that showed no abnormalities other than slightly lower-than-average intracranial volume.
    D. Fran's reported symptoms include hearing voices when she is upset or angry, fraught and intense relationships with peers, and a history of physical abuse and neglect. On mental status examinations, she has been noted to have a linear thought process.

3.   An 11-year-old girl is brought by her parents to your psychiatry clinic because she has had sudden onset of auditory hallucinations over the past 2 weeks. The parents deny any previous medical or psychiatric concerns and describe a happy, social child who is an average student in school. She is not taking any medications.

During the interview, you observe erratic shifts in her mental state and involuntary movements of her mouth and jaw. What is the likely cause of this patient's symptoms?

A. Childhood-onset schizophrenia.
B. Intoxication with older sibling's stimulant medication.
C. Anti-*N*-methyl-D-aspartate (NMDA) receptor encephalitis.
D. Major depressive disorder with psychotic features.

4.   EOS differs from adult-onset schizophrenia (AOS) in which of the following aspects?

A. EOS is diagnosed using different criteria than those used for AOS.
B. Neuroanatomical changes have been observed only in individuals with EOS.
C. Individuals with EOS have less severe negative symptoms.
D. Individuals with EOS are more likely to have premorbid histories of learning problems and/or motor abnormalities.

5.   Which of the following is true about most youth who report hearing voices?

A. They have schizophrenia.
B. They have bipolar disorder with psychosis.
C. They do not have a psychotic disorder.
D. They will eventually develop schizophrenia.

6.   On the basis of randomized controlled trials (RCTs), which of the following antipsychotic medications has demonstrated the best efficacy for schizophrenia in adolescents?

A. Ziprasidone.
B. Risperidone.
C. Asenapine.
D. Long-acting injectables.

7.   A large RCT that compared risperidone, olanzapine, and molindone for the treatment of EOS found which of the following?

A. Olanzapine and risperidone were superior to molindone in reducing psychotic symptoms.
B. Only 10% of youth continued their initial medication treatment for 52 weeks.
C. There were no differences in weight gain among the three study agents.
D. Molindone was superior to risperidone and olanzapine in reducing psychotic symptoms.

CHAPTER 19

Eating and Feeding Disorders

Kamryn T. Eddy, Ph.D.

1. A 15-year-old adolescent presents for an evaluation because of recent weight loss (he has fallen from the 25th to the 5th percentile for BMI). He expresses fear of weight gain and does not understand why his parents are bringing him in for an evaluation. His parents report that they see him eating large amounts of food after school, and they worry that he is making himself vomit. Which diagnosis best fits his presentation?

   A. Anorexia nervosa.
   B. Bulimia nervosa.
   C. Binge eating disorder.
   D. Atypical anorexia nervosa.

2. The three examples of rationales for food avoidance/restriction in avoidant/restrictive food intake disorder (ARFID) that are described in DSM-5 (American Psychiatric Association 2013) include which of the following?

   A. Lack of interest in eating or food, fear of weight gain, and fear of aversive consequences.
   B. Lack of interest in eating or food, binge eating, and sensory sensitivity.
   C. Sensory sensitivity, fear of aversive consequences, and lack of interest in eating or food.
   D. Sensory sensitivity, fear of weight gain, and lack of interest in eating or food.

3. Which of the following is suggested by family-based treatment for children and adolescents with anorexia nervosa and bulimia nervosa?

A. Dysfunctional family dynamics have contributed to the development of the eating disorder.
B. Parents must be included in the treatment because they are to blame for causing the eating disorder.
C. Parents are not to blame for causing the eating disorder and may actually be the child's best resource for achieving recovery.
D. Parents have very little idea how to refeed their child and typically need help from professionals.

4. Which of the following is assumed to be the core transdiagnostic mechanism that maintains eating disorders as viewed in cognitive-behavioral therapy for eating disorders?

A. Dieting.
B. Binge-eating/purging.
C. Childhood traumatic experience.
D. Overvaluation of body weight and shape.

5. Which of the following is true regarding psychopharmacology for eating disorders?

A. No medications are proven to treat anorexia nervosa.
B. Fluoxetine is the only FDA-approved medication available for the treatment of avoidant/restrictive food intake disorder.
C. Medications are not useful in the treatment of comorbidity in individuals with eating disorders.
D. Olanzapine is the first-line treatment for anorexia nervosa.

Reference

American Psychiatric Association: Diagnostic and Statistical Manual of Mental Disorders, 5th Edition. Arlington, VA, American Psychiatric Association, 2013

CHAPTER 20

Tic Disorders

Nicole Mavrides, M.D.

Nadina Abdullayeva, M.D.

1.   Which of the following is *false* regarding tics?

   A. Tics are distinguished by urges or sensations that precede the movements or sounds.
   B. Tics follow a specific rhythm and occur regularly in bouts.
   C. Tics may resolve over time.
   D. Complex motor tics can at times appear purposeful, like jumping or kissing.

2.   All of the following are modifiable risk factors for developing tics *except*

   A. Prematurity.
   B. Low birth weight.
   C. Maternal autoimmune disease.
   D. Family history of tics.

3.   Comorbidity with tic disorders and Tourette's disorder is extremely common. Which of these disorders is *not* frequently associated with tics?

   A. ADHD.
   B. Obsessive-compulsive disorder.
   C. Schizophrenia.
   D. Autism spectrum disorder.

4.	Which of the following is the most accurate statement regarding the course of tic disorders in an individual?

    A. If onset of tics is after age 8 years, the clinician must look elsewhere for the etiology of involuntary movements.
    B. Although psychosocial stressors such as teasing may worsen symptoms early on, studies show that these patients develop better coping skills and are more successful and resilient in the future.
    C. It is recommended that a person's tics be ignored in all settings; this helps the individual feel included and cared for during the distressing time of tics.
    D. Patients with tics or Tourette's disorder have four times the risk of suicide compared with the general population. The increase in risk remains substantial even after adjusting for psychiatric comorbidity.

5.	Eva, an 11-year-old girl, is brought to your office by her parents for evaluation of tics. As you converse with the parents, you observe both vocal and motor tics in Eva. She also frequently interrupts her parents with her own questions and walks around the office inquiring about posters. She jokes with her father and seems to be enjoying herself. You note that the parents seem uncomfortable with Eva's behavior and are trying to get her to sit quietly. Eva readily understands, apologizes for her behavior, and sits down. Which of the following would be your best next step?

    A. Eva's tics are obvious, likely causing significant distress. You should start an FDA-approved treatment immediately to help mitigate the social stigma she might be experiencing at school.
    B. Eva is clearly inattentive, intrusive, and hyperactive, and you likely will need to start a stimulant medication to help with her ADHD.
    C. You compliment the parents on having such a curious daughter and interview the family further to gather more information about all possible symptoms before prescribing anything.
    D. You recommend parent-child interaction therapy because the parents are clearly struggling with controlling their difficult child.

6.	Which of the following is true regarding the pharmacology of tic disorders?

    A. α-Agonists and dopamine blockers have shown equal efficacy in clinical practice, and the choice depends on the family's preference.
    B. The three FDA-approved medications (clonidine, guanfacine, and haloperidol) are the first-line treatment for any type of tics.
    C. Comprehensive Behavioral Intervention for Tics (CBIT) is the first-line recommended treatment for all tics before starting any medication.
    D. Depending on the nature of the tics, effects on quality of life, family resources, and much more, each patient's treatment should be approached on an individual basis, and pharmacology is not always the first step.

CHAPTER 2 1

Elimination Disorders

Wendy R. Martinez Araujo, M.D.

1. A 6-year-old boy has been receiving outpatient treatment for enuresis for the past 6 months. His parents ask if the problem will continue when he becomes a teenager. Which of the following statements is correct?

    A. There is a high rate of spontaneous remission of enuresis between ages 5 and 7 years and after age 12 years.
    B. Persistence of enuresis into late adolescence is common.
    C. There is a high rate of worsened symptoms around the time of puberty.
    D. If enuresis is treated, it will not persist.

2. A 7-year-old girl is brought to the pediatric clinic after she started wetting the bed over the past 4 months, indicating secondary enuresis. Which of the following is *not* a risk factor for secondary enuresis?

    A. A comorbid ADHD diagnosis.
    B. Family history of enuresis.
    C. Psychological stressors.
    D. Nonspecific behavioral disorder.

3. A 6-year-old girl who has been diagnosed with enuresis has tried various treatments without success. Of the listed medications, which would be the best option?

    A. Fluoxetine.
    B. Desvenlafaxine.
    C. Imipramine.
    D. Fluphenazine.

4.   What was the most significant side effect of the intranasal preparation of DDAVP, which led the FDA to issue a warning that the intranasal preparation should no longer be used for the treatment of primary nocturnal enuresis?

A. Epistaxis.
B. Headaches.
C. Hyponatremia.
D. Abdominal pain.

5.   A 7-year-old boy comes to the clinic accompanied by his mother. He started wetting the bed at night over the past 4 months. The mother is willing to start a behavioral treatment to stop bedwetting. What behavioral treatment has shown the same effectiveness as pharmacological treatment in enuresis?

A. Evening fluid restriction.
B. Retention-control training.
C. Reward system.
D. Bell and pad method of conditioning.

6.   A 6-year-old boy comes to the clinic, accompanied by his parent, with a history of 5 months of defecating in his clothes. The parent reports that the boy tends to have episodes of constipation for 2–3 days in a week and afterward will defecate in his clothes. What is the best behavior-based treatment for his presentation?

A. Bell and pad method conditioning.
B. Daily timed intervals on the toilet with rewards.
C. Evening restriction of food.
D. Encouragement to use the toilets at school.

CHAPTER 22

Sleep-Wake Disorders

Linda Schmidt, M.D.

1. With which of the following symptoms do children with narcolepsy usually present?

   A. Daytime sleepiness and sleep attacks.
   B. Excessive daytime sleepiness, cataplexy, hypnagogic hallucinations, and sleep paralysis.
   C. Excessive daytime sleepiness, hypnagogic hallucinations, and sleep paralysis.
   D. Excessive daytime sleepiness and sleep paralysis alternating with sleepwalking.

2. Which of the following psychiatric disorders has been found to have a strong association with restless legs syndrome (RLS) or periodic limb movement disorder (PLMD)?

   A. Generalized anxiety disorder.
   B. PTSD.
   C. ADHD.
   D. Autism spectrum disorder.

3. When is pharmacological treatment of RLS with iron supplementation usually recommended?

   A. When a child's serum ferritin level is below 25 ng/mL.
   B. When a child is diagnosed with RLS.
   C. When a child's serum ferritin level is below 50 ng/mL.
   D. When a child's serum ferritin level is between 80 and 100 ng/mL.

4. Which of the following is required to establish a diagnosis of obstructive sleep apnea (OSA) and to assess severity and treatment efficacy?

   A. Detailed sleep history and sleep diary.
   B. Nocturnal polysomnography (PSG).
   C. Diagnosis of adenotonsillar hypertrophy.
   D. Diagnosis of adenotonsillar hypertrophy and subsequent adenotonsillectomy.

5. Which of the following is recommended for children with OSA who either have not benefited from surgical intervention or are not candidates for surgery?

   A. Medication treatment (e.g., inhaled nasal steroids, antihistamines, nonsteroidal anti-inflammatory drugs)
   B. Continuous positive airway pressure (CPAP).
   C. Supplemental oxygen.
   D. Adenotonsillectomy.

6. Which of the following statements regarding parasomnias is true?

   A. They occur only during slow-wave sleep.
   B. They are much more frequently seen in adults than in children.
   C. They usually worsen during adolescence.
   D. They never cause sleep disruption.

7. Which of the following is the most common sleep-related symptom or condition in adolescents who use illicit drugs, alcohol, or cigarettes?

   A. Delayed sleep phase syndrome.
   B. Advanced sleep phase syndrome.
   C. Sleepwalking.
   D. Nightmares.

CHAPTER 23

Evidence-Based Practice

John Hamilton, M.D., M.Sc.
Eric Daleiden, Ph.D.
Eric Youngstrom, Ph.D.

1.   The base rate of a disorder used in Bayesian diagnostic approaches refers to which of the following?

A. The prevalence of the disorder in the population.
B. The prevalence of the disorder in the population adjusted for age and gender.
C. The prevalence of the disorder in the clinic population.
D. The lowest estimate of the disorder in the clinic population.

2.   According to Fixsen et al. (2005), which experience is essential for transferring skills from training experiences to patient interventions?

A. Studying recordings of oneself doing interventions with patients.
B. Supervision with experts trained in evidence-based treatment.
C. Peer supervision in a team setting led by an expert.
D. On-the-job coaching.

3.   Which of the following is not true regarding evidence-based practice (EBP)?

A. Even though EBP is a helpful tool, decisions about health care are based on the clinician's experience, regardless of the evidence base.
B. Decisions regarding treatment should be made by those receiving care, informed by the tacit and explicit knowledge of those providing care, within the context of available resources.

C. Loyalty to the status quo or use of merely available options, performed without measuring outcomes and implementation, is the opposite of EBP.

D. The singular term *evidence-based practice* refers to practice based on established processes for clinical decision making. The plural term *evidence-based practices* refers to those processes that are woven together to create EBP.

4. Which of the following is not in line with the principle of engaging patients and families with EBP?

A. Integrating evidence-based content into the initial contact between potential patients and care systems can create demand for EBPs and promote a match between patient characteristics and effective treatments.

B. Youth and families may help maintain EBPs by asking for and expecting services supported by evidence when they arrive at clinicians' offices.

C. The best way to engage patients and families is to not introduce EBP principles early because that may confuse them.

D. During orientation to clinical care, patients and families are encouraged to bring their own experiences and knowledge base to the evaluation process. This indicates respect for families as the experts on their own experiences, values, preferences, and history.

5. Which of the following is true regarding errors of commission and omission in the process of assessment?

A. Errors of commission assign invalid diagnoses. Errors of omission miss a diagnosis that should have been assigned.

B. Errors of commission miss a diagnosis, leading to no treatment of the true underlying condition. Errors of omission lead to a wrong diagnosis, leading to incorrect treatment.

C. When errors of commission occur, treatment may be provided without an appropriate informed consent process. Errors of omission refer to harm induced despite an informed consent process.

D. Errors of commission mean providing treatments that are not evidence-based and supported by research. Errors of omission mean not providing certain treatments despite the evidence.

Reference

Fixsen D, Naoom S, Blase K, et al: Implementation Research: A Synthesis of the Literature. Tampa, University of South Florida, 2005. Available at: https://nirn.fpg.unc.edu/sites/nirn.fpg.unc.edu/files/resources/NIRN-MonographFull-01-2005.pdf. Accessed August 11, 2020.

CHAPTER 24

Child Abuse and Neglect

Paramjit T. Joshi, M.D.

Lisa M. Cullins, M.D.

Anju Hurria, M.D., M.P.H.

1. A forensic evaluation of a child who has been physically or sexually abused should be performed by which of the following individuals?

   A. The child's therapist, who has experience with trauma-focused therapy.
   B. The child's pediatrician, who evaluates many children who have experienced abuse.
   C. The child's treating psychiatrist, whom the child sees once a month.
   D. A clinician trained in forensic assessments.

2. Which of the following factors might predict the degree of resilience in a child who has been abused?

   A. Interpersonal trust.
   B. Paternal conflicts.
   C. School violence.
   D. Living at home with parents.

3. Child abuse induces harm in many ways and can also be fatal. What is the leading cause of death in child abuse fatalities?

   A. Burns.
   B. Fracture.
   C. Head injury.
   D. Infection.

4. Characteristics of sexual abuse related to poor outcomes include which of the following?

   A. Longer duration, use of force, penetration, and a perpetrator who is close or related to the child.
   B. Longer duration, use of force, penetration, and a perpetrator who is a stranger.
   C. Shorter duration, use of force, penetration, and a perpetrator who is close or related to the child.
   D. Shorter duration, use of force, penetration, and a perpetrator who is a stranger.

5. Child neglect is a different issue from child abuse. Which of the following describes or indicates child neglect?

   A. The child has a nonaccidental injury.
   B. Responsible caretaking adults fail to provide adequate physical care and supervision.
   C. The child has been subjected to inappropriate physical touching.
   D. Abuse has been perpetrated on a teenager rather than a child.

6. Most experts believe that physical and sexual abuse result from a combination of factors that can be categorized into those related to families and those related to the child. Which of the following is a risk factor in the child that predisposes the child to being abused?

   A. Obesity.
   B. Educational status.
   C. Geographical location.
   D. Intellectual disability.

CHAPTER 25

Cultural and Religious Issues

Mary Lynn Dell, M.D., D.Min.

1. The term *ethnicity* refers to which of the following?

    A. The physical, biological, and genetic qualities of humans.
    B. An individual's spiritual and religious beliefs only.
    C. An individual's identity with a group of people sharing common origins, customs, and beliefs.
    D. The country of one's birth and its international political positions.

2. Which of the following best describes the concept of *religious fundamentalism*?

    A. Fluctuating beliefs of a spiritual nature, independent of the teachings, values, and behavioral expectations of specific religions and religious organizations.
    B. Strict interpretation of sacred writings and lifestyle practices guided by religious teachings that may be found worldwide in many major faith traditions.
    C. A philosophy of life that addresses life's most common, basic questions.
    D. Embracing modernity and new, popular spiritual concepts with enthusiasm.

3. A child and adolescent psychiatrist is caring for two different families who self-report membership and regular church attendance in the same Protestant denomination. One set of parents eschews premarital sex and all drug and alcohol use and insists that their children attend all of the youth activities at their church. The other set of parents states that they assume their children will be sexually active and use marijuana by the time they are in college. They permit an occasional beer on the weekends if their majority-age children will not be driving, and they did not enforce regular church attendance after their children reached high school. Which of the following is true about these families?

    A. The two families are an example of a continuum of beliefs and practices within the same and/or closely related religious denomination.

B. Families who have religious beliefs belong to organized religious communities, so there is no need for a mental health clinician to understand the role those beliefs and practices play in the value systems of the parents and individual adolescent children.

C. There is a possibility of emotional and/or physical neglect or abuse in the family that is more religiously observant and has stricter behavioral expectations for their children.

D. There is a possibility of emotional and/or physical neglect or abuse in the family that is less religiously observant and has more lenient behavioral expectations for their children

4. Which of the following is true regarding resources helpful for patients and families that are available through local religious institutions and faith-based organizations?

A. Child and adolescent psychiatrists should avoid collaborations with religious professionals, including hospital chaplains and clergy leaders in community churches, synagogues, mosques, and other houses of worship.

B. Religious/spiritual professionals and organizations have limited interest in medical care, health, and wellness, so there is no reason to seek resources for families from religious or faith-based organizations.

C. The need for assistance from faith-based organizations and religious communities has decreased greatly in recent years because health insurance and various secular treatment programs have multiplied and become less expensive.

D. Common resources available through religious groups and faith-based organizations include food pantries, clothes closets, shelters, health clinics, transportation to medical appointments, and daycare for young children.

5. The DSM-5 section "Cultural Formulation" (American Psychiatric Association 2013) includes which of the following?

A. Only a limited description of physical and emotional symptoms commonly experienced by refugees fleeing from specific countries.

B. No consideration of the ways suffering is communicated by individuals from diverse cultural groups.

C. Suggested outlines for inclusion of relevant information about cultural identity, cultural understandings of distress, psychosocial stressors and cultural features of vulnerability and resilience, and cultural understandings of the relationships between individuals and clinicians.

D. No information helpful for understanding children and adolescents younger than 18 years of age and their families.

C H A P T E R   2 6

Youth Suicide

David A. Brent, M.D.

Tina R. Goldstein, Ph.D.

Craig J.R. Sewall, Ph.D., LCSW

1. Sam, a 16-year-old boy, decides late one evening that he is going to kill himself to "end the pain." He grabs a bottle of pills from the bathroom and unscrews the cap, but before he is able to put any pills in his mouth, his mother knocks on the door. Sam puts the pills away and goes to bed. How should this event be classified?

    A. Suicide attempt.
    B. Interrupted suicide attempt.
    C. Aborted suicide attempt.
    D. Nonsuicidal self-injurious behavior.

2. Which of the following statements regarding suicidal thoughts and behaviors among male versus female youth is correct?

    A. The rate of death by suicide is higher for female youth than male youth.
    B. Male youth endorse higher rates of suicidal ideation than do female youth.
    C. The rate of attempted suicide is higher for female youth than male youth.
    D. Compared with cisgender youth, transgender youth are less likely to ideate and attempt suicide.

3. Approximately ____ of youth with suicidal ideation go on to attempt suicide.

    A. 50%.
    B. 10%.
    C. 25%.
    D. 33%.

4. Suicidal ideation should be assessed according to both severity (intent) and pervasiveness (frequency and intensity). Which of the following is *not* one of the four components of suicidal intent that should be explored?

    A. Extent to which the person wants to die.
    B. Preparatory behaviors.
    C. Prevention of discovery.
    D. Prior history of suicidal behavior .

5. Which of the following risk factors is the strongest predictor of future suicidal behavior?

    A. Previous self-injurious behavior.
    B. Having a mood disorder.
    C. Family history of suicidal behavior.
    D. Having a chronic medical condition.

6. All of the following are evidence-based approaches to clinical management of youth suicidality except

    A. Safety plans.
    B. Means restriction.
    C. Inpatient hospitalization.
    D. Cognitive-behavioral therapy.

CHAPTER 27

Gender and Sexual Diversity in Childhood and Adolescence

Jonathon Wanta, M.D.

Briahna Yuodsnukis, Ph.D.

Aron Janssen, M.D.

1. A 12-year-old nonbinary individual presents to your clinic for an initial assessment. They report 6 months of increasing anxiety and social isolation. Which of the following should be considered in assessing and formulating this patient?

    A. Bullying at school due to their nonbinary identity.
    B. Fear of rejection by friends and family.
    C. Baseline social anxiety.
    D. All of the above.

2. Which of the following describes how cumulative exposure to external stressors (such as bullying) and internal stressors (such as internalized homophobia) increases the risk of adverse mental and physical health outcomes?

    A. Minority stress theory.
    B. Transactional theory of stress and coping.
    C. Overcoming adversity theory.
    D. General adaptation syndrome.

3. Which of the following medical and surgical treatments is considered *fully reversible* for transgender and nonbinary youth?

    A. Puberty blockers.
    B. Gender-affirming testosterone therapy.
    C. Gender-affirming estrogen therapy.
    D. Vaginoplasty.

4. Most children can have a basic understanding of gender by what age?

    A. 1 year.
    B. 3 years.
    C. 7 years.
    D. 12 years.

5. Which of the following psychotherapeutic interventions is *not* recommended for transgender and gender nonbinary youth?

    A. Adapting evidence-based interventions to target minority stress sequelae.
    B. Cognitive-behavioral therapy (CBT) to change the patient's gender identity.
    C. Collaborating with and providing psychoeducation to families.
    D. Advocating for equitable and nondiscriminatory policies at school.

6. Which of the following questions is the most appropriate for assessing sexual orientation?

    A. Have you ever had a boyfriend?
    B. Are you romantically attracted to any peers at school?
    C. Are you romantically attracted to boys or girls?
    D. There is no need to ask because sexual minority patients will bring it up without prompting if it is important.

7. Which of the following publishes standards of care for clinicians in evaluating and managing transgender and gender-diverse individuals?

    A. The World Professional Association of Transgender Health (WPATH).
    B. The Trevor Project.
    C. The Family Acceptance Project.
    D. Parents, Families, and Friends of Lesbians and Gays (PFLAG).

CHAPTER 28

Aggression and Violence

Jeffrey H. Newcorn, M.D.

Yael Kufert, M.D.

Iliyan Ivanov, M.D.

Anil Chacko, Ph.D.

1. What is the relationship between alcohol and drug use disorders and aggression?

    A. Alcohol and drug use disorders are not associated with increased odds of aggression.
    B. Alcohol use disorder is not associated with increased odds of aggression, but drug use disorders are.
    C. Drug use disorders are not associated with increased odds of aggression, but alcohol use disorder is.
    D. Both alcohol use disorder and drug use disorders are associated with significantly increased odds of aggression toward self and others.

2. Which of the following statements regarding aggression and violence is the most accurate?

    A. Aggression and violence among youth are rare and do not represent a major public health concern.
    B. A temporary decrease in similar events often occurs over the 2 weeks following a mass school shooting.
    C. School shootings are less likely to occur in states with higher mental health expenditures.
    D. A temporary increase in similar events often occurs over the 2 months following a mass school shooting.

3. In neuroimaging studies, abnormal gray matter volumes in which of the following brain regions is found to be associated with aggressive behaviors?

    A. Ventral striatum.
    B. Insula.
    C. Dorsolateral prefrontal cortex.
    D. Cerebellum.

4. Which neurochemical has been associated with the development of antisocial personality disorder (ASPD) in late adolescence to early adulthood for boys?

    A. Dopamine.
    B. Testosterone.
    C. Serotonin.
    D. Glutamate.

5. Which of the following is true when more intensive antibullying programs are compared with less intensive ones?

    A. Both have similar outcomes.
    B. Better outcomes are found with more intensive programs.
    C. Poorer outcomes are found with more intensive programs.
    D. Insufficient data are available to compare varying intensities of antibullying programs.

6. A meta-analysis of studies of parent training programs (Wyatt Kaminski et al. 2008) found that all of the following are commonly used and effective aspects of parenting interventions for preventing aggressive behavior except

    A. Increasing positive parent-child interactions.
    B. Increasing parenting consistency.
    C. Behavioral reward systems.
    D. Problem-solving skills.

7. Which of the following statements regarding pharmacotherapy for aggressive behavior in children is correct?

    A. Treating underlying ADHD can be a useful strategy.
    B. No clinical trial data support the use of mood-stabilizing medications such as lithium and divalproex.
    C. Controlled clinical trials indicate that α_2-agonists effectively treat physical aggression in the context of ADHD.
    D. Risperidone is an FDA-approved treatment for aggression and should be the first medication used for this condition.

Reference

Wyatt Kaminski J, Valle LA, Filene JH, et al: A meta-analytic review of components associated with parent training program effectiveness. J Abnorm Child Psychol 36(4):567–589, 2008 18205039

CHAPTER 29

Psychiatric Emergencies

Lisa L. Giles, M.D.

1. Which of the following tools has been validated to screen for suicide risk in a pediatric emergency department (ED) setting?

    A. Suicide Assessment Five-Step Evaluation and Triage (SAFE-T).
    B. Ask Suicide-Screening Questions (ASQ).
    C. Patient Safety Screener (PSS-3).
    D. Patient Health Questionnaire–9 (PHQ-9).

2. A 14-year-old postmenarchal adolescent with a known history of anxiety and depression is brought to the ED by her parents after expressing suicidal ideation to her outpatient therapist. The patient denies any suicide attempts. A physical exam is normal with no obvious signs of toxicity. Which laboratory studies would be indicated during the assessment?

    A. Thyroid-stimulating hormone and free T_4.
    B. Complete blood count with differential, renal panel, and liver function tests.
    C. Pregnancy test.
    D. Erythrocyte sedimentation rate.

3. An ED crisis worker assesses a 16-year-old adolescent who is presenting to the ED after posting a suicide plan on his social media account. Which of the following features, if present in the patient's current presentation or history, would best support the consulting psychiatrist's recommendation for psychiatric hospitalization?

    A. The patient refuses to sign a no-suicide contract.
    B. The parents are requesting an admission.
    C. The patient is currently intoxicated.
    D. The patient describes a specific suicide plan with clear lethality and feasibility.

4. A 12-year-old boy is brought to the ED by the police after becoming aggressive at school. Which of the following should be included as part of the initial management in the emergency department?

   A. Administer intramuscular haloperidol and lorazepam.
   B. Place the patient in mechanical restraints.
   C. Provide a calm environment with preferred distractions while collecting additional history about triggers and helpful responses.
   D. Prepare for transfer for psychiatric hospitalization.

5. Which of the following is true regarding the use of antipsychotic medications to treat agitation in pediatric patients in the ED?

   A. Severe agitation, especially in the setting of delirium, psychosis, or alcohol intoxication, may indicate the use of antipsychotic medications.
   B. Combining intramuscular olanzapine with intravenous benzodiazepine when agitation is extreme is the ideal choice when medication use is necessary.
   C. Intravenous ziprasidone can be used to address extreme aggression.
   D. When agitation is escalating, it is appropriate to continue administering increasing dosages of antipsychotics.

6. The ED can be a particularly challenging environment for patients with autism spectrum disorder. Which of the following interventions may improve cooperation?

   A. Involve the primary caregiver when communicating and negotiating with the patient.
   B. Quickly introduce interventions to avoid increasing the patient's anticipatory anxiety.
   C. Encourage multiple staff members to check on the patient frequently.
   D. Place the patient in a room near the nurses' station so that the patient will be under constant observation and cannot leave the room for any reason.

7. A psychiatric consultation is requested for a 14-year-old female adolescent who presents in the ED with possible psychosis. In addition to the acute onset of hallucinations, she is observed to have waxing and waning levels of disorientation and agitation. Which of the following should be part of the management of this patient in the ED?

   A. Ensure that the patient's pain, if present, is adequately covered with opioid medications.
   B. Consider the use of lorazepam to help manage agitation.
   C. Immediately administer an antipsychotic and transfer the patient to a psychiatric hospital.
   D. Offer repeated reassurance and reorientation while evaluating the patient for underlying disease processes.

C H A P T E R   3 0

Family Transitions

Challenges and Resilience

Emanuel Martinez, M.D.

1.   When multistressed families are in therapy, which of the following is a concept that seeks to empower struggling families to master the challenges in their stress-laden lives?

   A. Resilience-oriented perspective.
   B. Problem-saturated family narrative.
   C. Problem-focused therapy.
   D. Strengths-oriented assessment.

2.   In Falicov's multilevel model for prevention and intervention with transnational families, which of the following refers to the relational context?

   A. The loss of social networks.
   B. Issues of cultural diversity.
   C. Reconstitution of old and new community bonds.
   D. Marital and parent-child interaction patterns.

3.   In divorce and stepfamily formation, what matters most for successful adaptation?

   A. Not having joint custody even when parents can cooperate.
   B. Parents staying together in an unhappy marriage rather than getting a divorce.
   C. The quality of relationships with parents and between parents.
   D. Receiving divorce mediation and collaborative counseling.

4. Which of these situations is an example of disenfranchised loss?

    A. Homicide.
    B. Miscarriage.
    C. Dementia.
    D. Fatal accident.

5. A 12-year-old girl recently lost her mother in a fatal car accident. The girl lives with her father, and the rest of the extended family lives out of state. As the mental health clinician for this family, which of the following should you recommend to minimize long-term complications associated with the loss of the mother?

    A. Mobilize the kin network.
    B. Minimize the meaning of loss.
    C. Suggest that the surviving parent remarry soon.
    D. Encourage the child to suppress her grief to support her father.

CHAPTER 31

Legal and Ethical Issues

Tapan Parikh, M.D., M.P.H.
Mina K. Dulcan, M.D.

1. Which of the following is true regarding the ethical principle of confidentiality when treating minors?

   A. The confidential information disclosed by a minor must be disclosed to a parent or guardian, and the minor should be informed of this.
   B. The confidential information disclosed by a minor must be disclosed to a parent or guardian; however, the minor does not need to be informed of this.
   C. The clinician should articulate the issues involved in confidentiality and informed consent as the treatment progresses. These are not important in the initial phase of treatment when rapport is still being built.
   D. This principle obligates the clinician to hold in confidence communications with the patient, even if a minor.

2. Which of the following is *not* in line with the regulatory guidance regarding the Health Insurance Portability and Accountability Act (HIPAA) from the U.S. Department of Health and Human Services?

   A. Unless a competent patient objects, the psychiatrist and other clinicians can speak with other family members assisting in the patient's treatment.
   B. When psychiatric disorder or substance abuse impairs a patient's capacities, mental health professionals may share patient-related information in the patient's best interest.
   C. Although the laws can vary from state to state, in no state can the laws regarding mental health confidentiality be stricter than the HIPAA regulations.
   D. Certain disclosures are permissible when patients present a serious and imminent threat to themselves or others.

3. Which of the following is *not* true regarding emancipated minors?

    A. Emancipated minors are generally older than age 15 years, living away from parents, and economically self-sufficient.
    B. Minors living with extended families or foster families are considered emancipated.
    C. Married minors are considered emancipated.
    D. Minors on active duty in the U.S. armed services are considered emancipated.

4. Which of the following is not part of the four elements of a professional negligence claim?

    A. Beneficence.
    B. Duty.
    C. Dereliction.
    D. Damages.

5. Which of the following accurately describes standards of evidence used in the legal system?

    A. The standard of a preponderance of the evidence (i.e., more likely than not) cannot be used in most civil proceedings.
    B. The highest standard of proof, "beyond a reasonable doubt," is required in cases where deprivation of fundamental rights or liberty is at stake, such as termination of parental rights.
    C. The intermediate standard of "clear and convincing evidence" is needed in juvenile court and delinquency proceedings.
    D. The highest standard of proof, "beyond a reasonable doubt," is used in criminal proceedings.

6. Child psychiatrists are increasingly being called on to testify as experts in various legal proceedings. Which of the following is true when the child and adolescent psychiatrist acts as an expert witness?

    A. The psychiatrist's opinion as an expert witness may ultimately result in harm to the child.
    B. Although a child psychiatrist who is acting as an expert witness does not usually function in a doctor-patient relationship in the case, some exceptions exist.
    C. When a psychiatrist is serving as an expert witness, the client is usually a parent or guardian.
    D. As an expert witness, the child psychiatrist writes a report, provides depositions, and/or testifies in court and may provide treatment recommendations to the patient's treating psychiatrist.

7. Which of the following is *not* an example of competence criteria that allow children to provide testimony?

   A. The capacity to register an event.
   B. The ability to accurately recall and recount the event.
   C. The capacity to communicate on the basis of suggestibility.
   D. The ability to distinguish truth from falsehood.

CHAPTER 32

Telemental Health and e-Mental Health Applications With Children and Adolescents

Ewa Bieber, M.D.

1.   Which of the following is a requirement under the Ryan Haight Online Pharmacy Consumer Protection Act of 2008?

   A. Pharmacies must keep a record of medications prescribed during telemental health visits.
   B. Controlled substances may not be prescribed during telemental health visits.
   C. Physicians must complete one in-person evaluation of the patient prior to prescribing a controlled substance.
   D. Patients using telemental health visits must fill prescriptions at online pharmacies.

2.   Through which of the following does the Centers for Medicare and Medicaid Services (CMS) define telemedicine as delivering health care services?

   A. A secure phone line.
   B. A real-time interactive conferencing system with audio.
   C. A real-time interactive videoconferencing system with both audio and video.
   D. A specific videoconferencing system licensed by the CMS.

3. Which of the following is *not* necessary during a telemental health visit?

   A. Modern, well-functioning equipment.
   B. Encrypted software.
   C. Consistent high-speed connectivity.
   D. The patient and the clinician must both be at a clinical site.

4. Which of the following is true regarding the documentation of a telemental health visit?

   A. A clear indication that the clinical visit was conducted through videoconferencing is a must, but it is not necessary to document the patient's and clinician's locations.
   B. The name of the videoconferencing system used must be documented.
   C. The patient's and clinician's locations during the visit need to be documented, but documenting a clear indication that the clinical visit was conducted through videoconferencing is optional.
   D. A clear indication that the clinical visit was conducted through videoconferencing and the locations of the patient and the clinician during the visit need to be documented.

5. Which of the following can be used to improve audio privacy during telemental health visits?

   A. Whispering.
   B. Encouraging patients to type sensitive information in the chat feature.
   C. Adding pillows to couches, curtains on windows, or tapestries on walls.
   D. Placing a white noise machine next to the videoconferencing equipment's speakers.

6. What contract between the health care entity and the internet vendor is required for telemedicine visits?

   A. The online telemedicine payment contract.
   B. The business associate agreement (BAA).
   C. The Health Insurance Portability and Accountability Act contract for telemedicine (HIPAA-CT).
   D. The managed care agreement.

C H A P T E R   3 3

Principles of Psychopharmacology

Esther S. Lee, M.D.
Robert L. Findling, M.D., M.B.A.

1.   Interviewing children can be more challenging compared with older adolescents or adults for all of the following reasons *except*

    A. Developmental variability in psychological and cognitive characteristics.
    B. Relative limitations in verbal abilities.
    C. More comfort and experience in recognizing emotions and feelings.
    D. Difficulty accurately estimating time increments.

2.   Preemptive cardiovascular risk stratification with a baseline electrocardiogram (ECG) may be important when considering higher-risk psychotropic medications, including all of the following *except*

    A. Lithium.
    B. First-generation antipsychotics.
    C. Carbamazepine.
    D. Tricyclic antidepressants.

3.   Pharmacokinetic differences between children and adults include all of the following *except*

    A. When adjusted for body weight, children may have proportionally more liver tissue than adults.
    B. Children may have proportionally more extracellular and total-body water than adults.

C. Children may have proportionally less fat tissue than adults.

D. Children may have lower glomerular filtration rates than adults when adjusted for body weight.

4. Which of the following federal legislative acts first gave pharmaceutical companies greater financial incentives to voluntarily conduct clinical trials of medications in children and adolescents?

A. The Pediatric Research Equity Act (PREA).

B. The U.S. Food and Drug Administration Modernization Act of 1997 (FDAMA).

C. The Best Pharmaceuticals for Children Act (BPCA).

D. The U.S. Food and Drug Administration Safety and Innovation Act.

5. All of the following reasons may contribute to treatment nonadherence to psychopharmacological treatment *except*

A. An authoritative communication style used by the clinician.

B. The emergence of adverse drug effects.

C. The social stigma associated with mental illness.

D. Pressure from family expectations or cultural beliefs.

CHAPTER 34

Medications Used for ADHD

Ronald Steingard, M.D.

Mark A. Stein, Ph.D.

John S. Markowitz, Pharm.D.

1. Which of the following options includes medications approved by the FDA for the treatment of ADHD?

    A. Methylphenidate, amphetamine, and bupropion.
    B. Guanfacine, amphetamine, and atomoxetine.
    C. Amphetamine, bupropion, and modafinil.
    D. Guanfacine, amphetamine, and modafinil.

2. Which of the following is true regarding treatment options for ADHD?

    A. Biological markers can be used to predict individual responses to ADHD treatments.
    B. Given the tolerability of stimulant medications, they can be started at the maximum recommended dose.
    C. Atomoxetine has been associated with initial weight loss.
    D. Bupropion, used off-label for ADHD, was originally developed as an antipsychotic.

3. Which of the following stimulant formulations has both a rapid onset of action and a brief duration of response?

    A. Concerta.
    B. Jornay PM.
    C. Evekeo.
    D. Mydayis.

4.   All of the following statements are true for the optimal treatment of ADHD with medication *except*

   A. Individualized dose titration is important.
   B. Routine monitoring using standard measures is necessary.
   C. Ongoing assessments should include observing for any side effects.
   D. Vital signs monitoring at baseline is necessary, but there is no need to monitor routinely.

5.   Which of the following statements is true regarding treatment adherence for ADHD in adolescents?

   A. Treatment adherence tends not to be an issue with standard treatment.
   B. Treatment adherence appears to be unrelated to concerns about stigma.
   C. Treatment adherence can be made worse by including the patient in treatment decisions.
   D. Treatment adherence can be improved with ongoing psychoeducation, medication adjustments, and shared decision-making.

6.   Which of the following is true regarding amphetamines?

   A. Amphetamines decrease the synaptic availability of dopamine and norepinephrine.
   B. Amphetamines hasten the reuptake of catecholamines from the synaptic cleft.
   C. Amphetamines increase the production of dopamine and norepinephrine.
   D. Amphetamines displace monoamines from intraneuronal storage vesicles.

7.   Cardiovascular effects of α_2-adrenergic receptor agonists include which of the following?

   A. Increased blood pressure.
   B. Decreased electrocardiogram PR interval.
   C. Decreased heart rate.
   D. Decreased ECG QTcF interval.

C H A P T E R   3 5

Antidepressants

Graham J. Emslie, M.D.
Jessica M. Jones, M.A.
Laura A. Stone, M.D.

1. Which of the following medications is *not* contraindicated in a patient taking a selective serotonin reuptake inhibitor (SSRI)?

   A. Pimozide.
   B. Selegiline.
   C. Trifluoperazine.
   D. Linezolid.

2. When considering the pharmacodynamics of antidepressants, what is unique about sertraline?

   A. It is the only SSRI with an affinity for dopamine receptors.
   B. At low dosages, it is primarily an SSRI. At higher dosages, it also acts as a norepinephrine reuptake inhibitor.
   C. It is the most potent serotonin and norepinephrine reuptake inhibitor among the SSRIs.
   D. It inhibits the reuptake of norepinephrine and dopamine.

3. Which atypical antidepressant (non-SSRI) has received approval from the FDA for use in youth?

   A. Mirtazapine.
   B. Bupropion.
   C. Trazodone.
   D. Duloxetine.

4. Which two antidepressants have received approval from the FDA for the treatment of depression in adolescents?

   A. Citalopram and escitalopram.
   B. Escitalopram and fluoxetine.
   C. Fluoxetine and fluvoxamine.
   D. Paroxetine and sertraline.

5. Which SSRI that may be used for the treatment of OCD in youth is more likely to cause discontinuation symptoms due to its short half-life?

   A. Fluoxetine.
   B. Fluvoxamine.
   C. Paroxetine.
   D. Sertraline.

6. Which of the following atypical antidepressants is a nonselective N-methyl-D-aspartate (NMDA) antagonist?

   A. Bupropion.
   B. Ketamine.
   C. Levomilnacipran.
   D. Vortioxetine.

7. When does antidepressant-induced activation typically emerge?

   A. On discontinuation of the medication.
   B. When the maximum recommended dosage is exceeded.
   C. On achieving a steady state of medication.
   D. Early in treatment or following a dosage increase.

CHAPTER 36

Mood Stabilizers

Courtney Heim, D.O.

1. Which of the following is true regarding lithium treatment for bipolar disorder?

   A. Serious neurological symptoms such as seizures, coma, and death can occur when lithium level is above 2 mEq/L.
   B. Lithium is FDA approved for the treatment of acute manic and mixed states in patients ages 7 years and older as monotherapy and maintenance treatment of bipolar I disorder.
   C. Baseline electrocardiogram (ECG) is not necessary with lithium treatment initiation.
   D. Diabetes insipidus is an irreversible adverse effect following lithium use.

2. A 15-year-old male adolescent with a past psychiatric history of bipolar disorder is seen in the clinic for follow-up. His mood has been stable on lamotrigine for years. However, he was recently hospitalized because of increasingly severe aggression, and another medication was prescribed to target the aggression. The lamotrigine dosage was unchanged when this new medication was added. Unfortunately, the patient developed erythematous desquamative lesions all over his body, including severe oral ulcers. What is the most likely medication that was started during his hospitalization?

   A. Quetiapine.
   B. Amitriptyline.
   C. Lithium.
   D. Valproate.

3.   Which medication would be contraindicated in a person with HLA-B gene variant *HLA-B*1502*?

A. Lithium.
B. Lamotrigine.
C. Carbamazepine.
D. Gabapentin.

4.   A 17-year-old female adolescent was started on lamotrigine as a maintenance medication to prevent future mood episodes. A new medication was added, and shortly afterward, she had a reoccurrence of depressive symptoms. What medication was likely added?

A. Valproate.
B. Carbamazepine.
C. Lithium.
D. Topiramate.

5.   Oxcarbazepine is structurally related to carbamazepine—that is, oxcarbazepine is the 10-keto analogue of carbamazepine. Which of the following is true regarding differences between clinical use of carbamazepine and oxcarbazepine?

A. Both carbamazepine and oxcarbazepine carry FDA-approved indications for acute manic and mixed episodes in bipolar I disorder in adults.
B. Carbamazepine is indicated by the FDA for the treatment of partial seizures but not generalized tonic seizures, and the same is true for oxcarbazepine.
C. Although oxcarbazepine has an FDA indication for the treatment of certain mood episodes in adults with bipolar I disorder, carbamazepine does not have any evidence base for the treatment of bipolar disorder.
D. Although carbamazepine has an FDA indication for the treatment of certain mood episodes in adults with bipolar I disorder, oxcarbazepine does not have any evidence base for the treatment of bipolar disorder.

CHAPTER 37

Antipsychotic Medications

Abdullah Bin Mahfodh, M.D.

1. Which of the following is correct regarding cytochrome P450 (CYP) enzymes and the metabolism of antipsychotics?

   A. CYP3A4 is a low-affinity, high-capacity enzyme most relevant in the metabolism of aripiprazole, iloperidone, perphenazine, and risperidone.
   B. CYP2D6 is a high-affinity, low-capacity enzyme most relevant in the metabolism of clozapine and olanzapine.
   C. CYP1A2 is a low-affinity, high-capacity enzyme that is relevant for the clearance of clozapine and, to some degree, olanzapine.
   D. CYP2C19 and 2C9 are relevant only for risperidone clearance.

2. Which of the following antipsychotics is approved by the FDA for Tourette's disorder in children and adolescents?

   A. Quetiapine.
   B. Olanzapine.
   C. Brexpiprazole.
   D. Aripiprazole.

3. Tardive dyskinesia is less prevalent in youth than in adults, but it can significantly affect the quality of life and should be appropriately addressed immediately. Which of the following is *not* one of the strategies to address tardive dyskinesia?

   A. Add vitamin B_{12}.
   B. Reduce the dosage of antipsychotic medication.
   C. Add vitamin E.
   D. Increase the dosage of antipsychotic medication (masking).

4. Which of the following is true regarding side effects of antipsychotic medications in children and adolescents?

 A. All antipsychotic medications are associated with a risk of developing myocarditis.
 B. Children and adolescents are less sensitive than adults to extrapyramidal side effects (EPS) associated with first-generation antipsychotics (FGAs) and second-generation antipsychotics (SGAs).
 C. Withdrawal dyskinesia rates appear to be higher with SGAs than FGAs.
 D. The weight gain potential of SGAs follows roughly the same rank order as in adults, but the magnitude is greater.

5. When prescribing antipsychotics, adverse effect assessment and monitoring should be proactive, considering developmental norms and thresholds. All of the following should be monitored or assessed routinely in children and adolescents taking antipsychotic medications *except*

 A. Serum fasting blood glucose (or hemoglobin A1C).
 B. Weight and height (calculate BMI percentile and BMI z-score).
 C. Parkinsonism and akathisia.
 D. Serum prolactin.

6. Which of the following is an example of a primary prevention strategy for youth treated with antipsychotic medications?

 A. Intensifying healthy lifestyle instructions in overweight patients and those with mild baseline metabolic abnormalities, significant weight gain, or beginning metabolic abnormalities during therapy.
 B. Choosing an agent with the lowest likelihood of adverse effects on body composition and metabolic status.
 C. Intensifying weight reduction interventions in patients who are obese or have clinically defined related abnormalities.
 D. Consideration of switching to a lower-risk agent in overweight patients and those with mild baseline metabolic abnormalities, significant weight gain, or beginning metabolic abnormalities during treatment.

7. Antipsychotics may prolong QTc interval. Which of the following is *not* true regarding obtaining a baseline electrocardiogram (ECG)?

 A. Obtain an ECG if there is a family history of early sudden death or prolonged QT syndrome.
 B. Obtain an ECG if there is a personal history of irregular heartbeat, unexplained tachycardia, or shortness of breath at rest.
 C. Because there is a significantly higher risk of QTc prolongation in children and adolescents, an ECG should ideally be obtained at baseline.
 D. Obtain an ECG if there is a personal history of dizziness on exertion or syncope.

CHAPTER 38

Individual Psychotherapy

Jonathon Pochyly, Ph.D.

1. Which of the following terms implies spoken verbal interventions by the therapist commenting on a child's psychological conflicts?

    A. Clarification.
    B. Interpretations.
    C. Reenactment.
    D. Mentalization.

2. It is important for a child psychotherapist to include all of the following in any psychotherapy with children *except*

    A. A flexible approach to the therapy.
    B. Awareness of cultural differences in the child's background.
    C. Encouraging a healthy transference of old attitudes to the therapist.
    D. Adjustments to meet the child's level of understanding.

3. Which of the following is considered a working psychological explanation of the patient's feelings, behaviors, and thinking?

    A. Assessment.
    B. Diagnosis.
    C. Formulation.
    D. Conceptualization.

4. Which of the following is most likely not very useful or effective in therapy when a child is not talking much in the early sessions?

    A. Asking questions about the child's life.
    B. Sitting quietly with the child so that they can feel empowered to talk.

C. Talking at length about video games the child might be playing at home.

D. Playing a game that does not require any talking.

5. The role of parents in the child's individual psychotherapy can be varied but should always include which of the following?

A. Informing the parent(s) of what is troubling their child.

B. Discussing with the parent(s) the potential impact of significant events in the session.

C. The therapist being conscientious and thorough in deciding what to share with the parent(s).

D. The parent having ongoing awareness of the goals and progress of the therapy.

6. The following are important and helpful considerations when terminating therapy with a child *except*

A. Taking into consideration whether the primary and secondary goals of treatment have been met.

B. Tapering the frequency of therapy sessions leading to termination.

C. Discussing termination when the family feels that the child has shown improvement.

D. Avoiding providing occasional booster sessions because this may be confusing to the child.

CHAPTER 39

Parent Counseling, Psychoeducation, and Parent Support Groups

Jennifer B. Reese, Psy.D.
Mary A. Fristad, Ph.D., ABPP

1. The term *psychoeducation* refers to a wide range of interventions. Psychoeducation initially emerged to improve the prognosis of which disorder?

    A. Bipolar disorder.
    B. Anorexia nervosa.
    C. Selective mutism.
    D. Schizophrenia.

2. Which of the following terms refers to the type and quality of family members' interactions and attitudes regarding a person who has a mental illness?

    A. Emotional energy.
    B. Emotional intelligence.
    C. Expressed emotion.
    D. Ego explanation.

3. Which of the following can be targets or topics of multifamily psychoeducational psychotherapy (MF-PEP) for both children and parents?

    A. Medications, problem-solving skills, and mood disorders and family life.
    B. Medications, systems of care, and communication.

C. Medications, symptom management techniques, and systems of care.

D. Medications, problem-solving skills, and communication.

4. Compared with a wait list control group, youth in a study who received MF-PEP experienced which of the following?

A. No change in mood symptoms.

B. Worsening of mood symptoms.

C. Decrease in mood symptom severity.

D. Remission of mood symptoms.

5. All of the following reflect responsibilities of a support group facilitator *except*

A. Allowing participants to share whatever is troubling them.

B. Managing logistics.

C. Creating a safe environment.

D. Referring members to resources.

CHAPTER 40

Behavioral Parent Training

Melissa R. Dvorsky, Ph.D.
Amanda Steinberg, B.S.

1.   A parent engages in "special time" with their son by putting together a puzzle. The child attempts to fit an edge piece into the center. What should the parent do in response?

    A. Let the child figure out where the puzzle piece fits on his own.
    B. Ask the child questions about the puzzle piece to provide guidance.
    C. Hand the child another piece and explain why it fits better.
    D. Redirect the child to start with an easier section of the puzzle.

2.   Which of the following is *not* recommended for monitoring treatment progress in behavioral parent training?

    A. The clinician asks parents, "What rewards did your child earn and how often?"
    B. The clinician reviews the child's home behavior chart or daily report card data.
    C. The clinician observes parent-child interactions in a clean-up activity.
    D. The clinician rates their perception of parent engagement.

3.   A mother is finishing dinner at home when her son, Dillon, begins to throw a tantrum. Exhausted from her day at work, the mother tries to get Dillon to quiet down quickly, saying she will give him a dessert if he calms down. Dillon stops and is provided dessert. What will this situation likely result in?

    A. An increase in tantrums.
    B. A decrease in tantrums.
    C. A static trend in tantrums.
    D. There is not enough information to determine the future trend of Dillon's tantrums.

4. Mrs. Adams is on her third week of using a token economy reward system with her son, Ben. Ben struggles with getting his homework done after school, so his goal is to complete his homework before 4:00 P.M. with no more than one reminder. Ben fulfilled his homework routine after school in the first week to earn all points on his behavioral reward chart. However, in the second and third weeks, Mrs. Adams had to give multiple reminders, and he earned his daily reward only once. Ben and his mother are frustrated, and Ben repeatedly complains that the behavioral reward chart is not going to work. What would be the most appropriate next step for Mrs. Adams to address this?

    A. Stop implementing the token economy and consider other behavioral parenting strategies.
    B. Restate to Ben what his goals are and see how he responds.
    C. Increase the criterion from one reminder for completing his homework to two or three reminders.
    D. Do nothing and allow more time for Ben to adjust to the new system.

5. Which of the following factors is least likely to influence behavioral intervention treatment outcomes?

    A. Parents with low socioeconomic status.
    B. The number of children in a family.
    C. Single-parent families.
    D. Parents who believe that their child is behaving badly on purpose.

6. The triad of disorders identified as disruptive behavior disorders that behavioral parent training was developed to address most commonly includes the following DSM-5 (American Psychiatric Association 2013) diagnoses *except* which of the following?

    A. ADHD.
    B. Oppositional defiant disorder.
    C. OCD.
    D. Conduct disorder.

Reference

American Psychiatric Association: Diagnostic and Statistical Manual of Mental Disorders, 5th Edition. Arlington, VA, American Psychiatric Association, 2013

CHAPTER 41

Family-Based Assessment and Treatment

Karen R. Gouze, Ph.D.
Richard Wendel, Ph.D.

1. A 5-year-old boy, accompanied by his parents, presents in your office with several symptoms, including temper tantrums, high levels of negative affect, and reluctance to attend school. All of the following would be the benefits of family therapy *except*

   A. Improved parenting skills.
   B. Reduction in symptoms.
   C. Parent satisfaction with the treatment.
   D. Improvement in symptoms of ADHD.

2. Which of the following options is a more important focus in family therapy than in individual therapy?

   A. The child's symptoms.
   B. The parent's symptoms.
   C. Patterns of interaction that create or contribute to the child's symptoms.
   D. Normal developmental processes.

3. Which of the following is an important family variable that contributes to externalizing behavior in children?

   A. Clear parental boundaries.
   B. Parental hostility.
   C. Sibling rivalry.
   D. Living with extended family members.

4.   A family comes to your office for the treatment of their 14-year-old son. When you ask what brings them to therapy, they launch into a long list of grievances about their child, including his substance use, disrespect, failing grades, and use of unacceptable language. In family therapy, this presentation is considered to be which of the following?

A. A problem-saturated narrative.
B. A family-based description of the problem.
C. A contextually sensitive narrative.
D. A well-formulated problem description.

5.   Which of the following is *not* part of the family therapy technique known as *joining*?

A. Avoid the "What's wrong?" question.
B. Start with relationship-building small talk with each person in the room.
C. Avoid talking about serious problems until everyone has a chance to connect with the therapist.
D. Immediately discuss the serious issues as soon as they are talked about, even if everyone in attendance has not had a chance to enter the process.

6.   Integrative Module-Based Family Therapy (IMBFT) is best described as which of the following?

A. An integrative approach to family therapy.
B. A psychoanalytic approach to family therapy.
C. A cognitive-behavioral approach to family therapy.
D. A psychiatric/biological approach to family therapy.

7.   *Reframing* is a technique used in which of the following domains of IMBFT?

A. The attachment/relationship domain.
B. The mastery domain.
C. The cognitive/narrative domain.
D. The affect regulation domain.

CHAPTER 42

Interpersonal Psychotherapy for Depressed Adolescents

Meredith L. Gunlicks-Stoessel, Ph.D.
Laura Mufson, Ph.D.

1. The therapist explains to an adolescent with depression and her parents that it is important for the teen to do as many of her activities as possible, such as getting to school, doing homework, and participating in after-school activities, but with the awareness and acceptance that the teen might not do these things as often or as well as before the depression developed. What is this explanation called?

    A. Behavioral activation.
    B. Cognitive restructuring.
    C. Increasing pleasurable activities.
    D. Limited sick role.

2. Which of the following describes the closeness circle in interpersonal psychotherapy?

    A. It is helpful in the middle phase to assist in role-play.
    B. It is used to identify relationships and guide the interpersonal inventory.
    C. It illustrates how the adolescent's depression symptoms affect their relationships.
    D. It is completed as part of homework in the initial phase of treatment.

3. A teenage girl became depressed after her mother's remarriage, their subsequent move to a new community, and the inclusion of stepsisters in the home. She and her mother have not been getting along well since the move. Which of the follow-

ing is the best description of her struggles according to the interpersonal psycho-therapy model?

A. Grief.
B. Interpersonal deficits.
C. Interpersonal role disputes.
D. Interpersonal role transitions.

4. Which of the following is *not* a goal for the problem area of interpersonal role disputes?

A. Gain interpersonal problem-solving skills to resolve the dispute.
B. Identify the teen's expectations for the other person and the other person's expectations for the teen.
C. Mourn the loss of how the relationship used to be.
D. Gain communication skills to resolve the dispute.

5. All of the following techniques are used in interpersonal psychotherapy for depressed adolescents (IPT-A) *except*

A. Communication analysis.
B. Cognitive restructuring.
C. Role-playing.
D. Decision analysis.

6. Which of the following is not one of the tasks for the termination phase of treatment with interpersonal psychotherapy?

A. Share feelings about ending the relationship with the therapist.
B. Review strategies that were practiced during treatment.
C. Review warning signs of depression.
D. Review mood ratings and events that could affect mood ratings in the future.

CHAPTER 43

Cognitive-Behavioral Treatment for Anxiety and Depression

Ashley Winch, M.S.

1. Why is parental involvement in cognitive-behavioral therapy (CBT) an integral part of treatment?

   A. Parental involvement in treatment aids in the development of appropriate goals for treatment.
   B. Parental involvement in treatment aids in the teaching and implementation of the skills learned in treatment.
   C. Parental involvement in treatment can lead to more effective parenting practices that can increase the likelihood of remission.
   D. All of the above.

2. A 12-year-old patient begins treatment for injection phobia. You determine that CBT is the optimal treatment method for this youth. Because of his fear of being given an injection, the patient has such intense anxiety that he refuses to leave the house if he is aware that there will be a doctor's appointment. What would be a potentially appropriate early step in a graduated exposure for this patient?

   A. Relaxation training.
   B. Showing him a picture of someone like him receiving an injection.
   C. Teaching him how to engage in cognitive restructuring.
   D. Driving him to the doctor's office without telling him where he is going.

3. Social skills training may be an important component of CBT for children and adolescents in treatment for which of the following?

    A. Depression but not social anxiety.
    B. Generalized anxiety without social anxiety.
    C. Social anxiety but not depression.
    D. Depression or social anxiety.

4. With regard to mood monitoring as an intervention for a child or an adolescent with depression, which of the following is beneficial for them to monitor?

    A. Any of their negative moods.
    B. Their negative and positive moods.
    C. Their depression-related moods.
    D. Their depression- or anxiety-related moods.

5. The Child/Adolescent Anxiety Multimodal Study (CAMS; Walkup et al. 2008) was a randomized controlled trial that examined the efficacy of CBT, pharmacological intervention, a combination of CBT and pharmacological intervention, and pill placebo for children and adolescents with anxiety. The Treatment for Adolescents With Depression Study (TADS; March et al. 2004; Treatment for Adolescents With Depression Study Team 2003) used the same model to determine the efficacy of these treatments in adolescents with depression. Which of the following accurately describes the findings from these studies?

    A. The combination of CBT and pharmacological intervention resulted in the highest remission rates.
    B. Pharmacological intervention resulted in the highest remission rates.
    C. The combination of CBT and pharmacological intervention resulted in the highest initial remission rates.
    D. CBT intervention resulted in the highest remission rates.

References

March J, Silva S, Petrycki S, et al: Fluoxetine, cognitive-behavioral therapy, and their combination for adolescents with depression: Treatment for Adolescents With Depression Study (TADS) randomized controlled trial. JAMA 292(7):807–820, 2004 15315995

Treatment for Adolescents With Depression Study Team: Treatment for Adolescents With Depression Study (TADS): rationale, design, and methods. J Am Acad Child Adolesc Psychiatry 42(5):531–542, 2003 12707557

Walkup JT, Albano AM, Piacentini J, et al: Cognitive behavioral therapy, sertraline, or a combination in childhood anxiety. N Engl J Med 359(26):2753–2766, 2008 18974308

CHAPTER 44

Motivational Interviewing

Kelly Walker Lowry, Ph.D.

1. All of the following are true regarding motivational interviewing (MI) *except*

   A. According to a meta-analysis, 75% of participants benefit from MI.
   B. MI has a proven role in treating youth substance use and youth with psychiatric comorbidities.
   C. MI has known utility in pediatric behavioral health concerns, including in patients with diabetes or asthma.
   D. MI studies have found larger effect sizes with ethnic majority youth compared with minority youth.

2. According to the MI model, which of the following terms describes the concept that the therapist and client are equal experts?

   A. Acceptance.
   B. Compassion.
   C. Partnership.
   D. Evocation.

3. Which of the following options correctly describes OARS, the four MI processes?

   A. Optimism, adaptations, reflections, and summaries.
   B. Open-ended questions, affirmations, reflections, and summaries.
   C. Object relations, affirmations, reflections, and summaries.
   D. Open-ended questions, adaptations, responsiveness, and summaries.

4. Which of the following is true regarding MI?

   A. MI is an example of an unstructured psychotherapy approach.
   B. It is best not to combine MI with other approaches such as cognitive-behavioral therapy (CBT).
   C. MI can be learned and competently practiced by clinicians from various disciplines.
   D. MI requires highly specialized training that is not available to some disciplines.

5. Which of the following is true regarding MI and group treatment?

   A. MI should not be used as a group treatment at any age.
   B. MI is effective in group treatment settings, including youth group treatment.
   C. MI can be used as a group treatment with no distinction from other approaches for group treatment.
   D. It is crucial for group members to demonstrate readiness for change for effective MI delivery.

C H A P T E R   4 5

Systems of Care, Wraparound Services, and Home-Based Services

Yann B. Poncin, M.D.

1.   Which of the following best describes wraparound services?

A. Wraparound services are a process for engaging with families to bring to-gether an array of informal and formal community services to support the needs of a child and family.
B. Wraparound services are a primary tool for engaging with families in Multi-systemic Therapy (MST).
C. Wraparound services are one of the four domains of clinical care used by In-tensive In-Home Child and Adolescent Psychiatric Services (IICAPS).
D. Wraparound services describes intakes conducted in which caregivers and other adults involved in a child's life are interviewed.

2.   What is the system of care (SOC)?

A. The SOC refers to the school, child protection, judicial, and mental health treatment services within a given community.
B. The SOC comprises the informal and formal supports available in a given community, including as an integral part the linkage of supports and coordi-nating access to care.
C. The SOC describes the federal, state, county, and local mental health service system and its coordination.
D. The SOC represents the formal and informal support services that are coordi-nated across tribal organizations in the United States.

3. Each of the following options is a key feature of home-based or intensive home-based services *except*

   A. 24-hour availability (24/7).
   B. Services delivered in the community.
   C. Psychiatric care.
   D. Small caseloads.

4. Which of the following acts or programs is not related to the emerging provision of mental health care for children?

   A. Mental Retardation Facilities and Community Mental Health Centers Construction Act.
   B. Child and Adolescent Service System Program.
   C. Comprehensive Community Mental Health Services for Children and Their Families Program.
   D. Individuals with Disabilities Education Act.

5. What was the intent of the Adoption Assistance and Child Welfare Act of 1980?

   A. To provide better funding for foster care agencies.
   B. To ameliorate the conditions in which children live before placement.
   C. To provide better funding for foster care parents.
   D. To strengthen permanency planning for children.

CHAPTER 46

Milieu Treatment

Inpatient, Partial Hospitalization, and Residential Programs

Khushbu Shah, M.D., M.P.H.

1. What is the best way to prevent elopement and risky behaviors in milieu treatment programs?

    A. Effective communication.
    B. Smaller unit census.
    C. Active parental involvement in treatment.
    D. Availability of PRN medications.

2. Readmission rate is one of the quality measures for inpatient units according to the Centers for Medicare and Medicaid Services and the Affordable Care Act. Return to hospitalization in which one of the following time frames defines readmission?

    A. 24 hours.
    B. 48 hours.
    C. 30 days.
    D. 60 days.

3. Which of the following factors is associated with a lower rehospitalization rate?

    A. Longer inpatient hospitalization stays.
    B. Longer period of day treatment.
    C. Younger age of the patient.
    D. Use of psychotropic medications.

4.   Carter, a 14-year-old adolescent, presents with a history of depression and anxiety, with worsening symptoms in the context of several psychosocial stressors at home and school. His home environment is currently unstable, and his aunt, his primary caregiver, has recently needed to take on a second job because of financial stressors. Carter's aunt has not been able to provide consistent supervision for medication monitoring or take him to therapy appointments. In the past, Carter has decompensated when he was nonadherent to treatment recommendations or did not have close structure and supervision. He currently denies active suicidal ideation or self-injurious behaviors but has recently had some thoughts and urges. Which of the following is the most appropriate placement?

   A. Acute inpatient psychiatric unit.
   B. Partial hospitalization program.
   C. Therapeutic day school.
   D. Residential treatment center.

5.   Which of the following is one of the two most common types of therapeutic modalities applied in therapeutic milieus?

   A. Dialectical behavioral therapy (DBT).
   B. Motivational interviewing (MI).
   C. Interpersonal psychotherapy (IPT).
   D. Parent management training (PMT).

CHAPTER 47

School-Based Interventions

Erika Ryst, M.D.

Jeff Q. Bostic, M.D., Ed.D.

Sharon A. Hoover, Ph.D.

Kris Scardamalia, Ph.D., LSSP, LP

1. All of the following are components of a comprehensive school mental health program *except*

    A. Psychiatric medication management services delivered in the school setting.
    B. Collaboration between school and community partners.
    C. Mental health screening, early identification of problems, and triage to appropriate levels of support.
    D. Multitiered evidence-based interventions to promote mental health.

2. Which of the following is true regarding a Section 504 plan that is generated by a school for a student?

    A. It enables the student to receive classroom accommodations by regular education staff.
    B. It provides specialized instruction for the student.
    C. It modifies the curriculum by lowering academic standards.
    D. It provides the same legal protections as an individualized education program (IEP).

3. A child psychiatrist is a consultant for her local school district and also provides direct services to students within the school. One of her direct service patients is

not receiving needed speech therapy services that are listed on the patient's IEP. What should the child psychiatrist do when addressing this issue?

A. Clarify that her primary role for this case is as the child's provider.
B. Respect the fact that it is up to the school's discretion to follow her suggestions.
C. Work with administrative staff to develop quality control procedures that ensure that all IEPs are implemented correctly.
D. Leave it to the child's pediatrician to advocate for the child's school services in order to avoid a conflict of interest.

4. Which of the following best describes the role of a school psychologist?

A. The majority of their time is spent conducting psychological assessments.
B. They are the primary providers of psychosocial interventions in schools.
C. They assist students in college or vocational planning and academic planning.
D. They act as a liaison between the school and the community.

5. Bounce Back is a targeted small-group school-based intervention for at-risk students with symptoms of which of the following?

A. Trauma.
B. Anxiety.
C. Depression.
D. Substance misuse.

6. A psychiatrist is asked to consult on a fifth-grade student with a learning disorder and ADHD. The teacher reports that the student repeatedly gets out of his seat and distracts the class with jokes when the class is asked to read independently and silently. The teacher is frustrated because she has redirected the student from this behavior numerous times without effect. She says, "I just want to find some strategies that will get him to stop disrupting the class." Which of the following consultation tactics would be most useful for the psychiatrist to employ at this time?

A. Suggest that the student may be using these behaviors to distract from the fact that he struggles with reading.
B. Praise the teacher for her perseverance in repeatedly redirecting the student.
C. Backtrack to the teacher's original intention to improve the students' reading skills.
D. Use the teacher's own words, "strategies that will get him to stop disrupting the class," to frame the intervention.

7. According to the University of Virginia's Comprehensive School Threat Assessment Guidelines, which of the following indicates that the school can likely screen out a threat as transient?

A. When the threat is an expression of humor, anger, or frustration.
B. When the threat includes a detailed plan to harm.

C. When the threat involves peers in the planning.
D. When the threat includes proclamations such as "something big will happen next week."

C H A P T E R   4 8

Collaborating With Primary Care

Elise Fallucco, M.D.

Rachel Ballard, M.D., M.A.

1. Which of the following is the largest benefit of integrated or collaborative care models compared with traditional outpatient care?

   A. Integrated or collaborative care models enable child and adolescent psychiatrists (CAPs) to provide long-term care for patients in pediatric settings.
   B. Reimbursement is higher for clinical services in an integrated or collaborative care model.
   C. Integrated or collaborative care models facilitate treatment for a larger population of youth.
   D. Patients with severe, complex psychopathology can be managed in a pediatric setting using integrated or collaborative care models.

2. Who serves as the director of the care team in the University of Washington AIMS Center model of collaborative care?

   A. The child and adolescent psychiatrist.
   B. The primary care provider.
   C. The behavioral health care coordinator.
   D. The parent(s) or caregiver(s) of the child.

3.	Which of the following distinguishes the consultative collaboration model from child psychiatry access programs?

A. The consultative collaboration model allows psychiatrists to care for a larger population than is typically served by child psychiatry access programs.
B. The consultative collaboration model is often supported by state-level funding.
C. The consultative collaboration model provides primarily same-day telephone consultation.
D. The consultative collaboration model allows psychiatrists to personally examine patients and provide a higher level of consultation.

4.	Which of the following strategies can facilitate primary care clinician engagement in collaborative care models?

A. Identify champions within the pediatric practice.
B. Implement training in a convenient and accessible format for clinicians.
C. Develop a plan for ongoing consultation.
D. All of the above.

5.	In models of collaborative care in which a mental health clinician has not directly evaluated the patient, what is the most appropriate way to give recommendations?

A. "In cases like these, we generally titrate the antidepressant if there has been minimal improvement after 4 weeks."
B. "For this patient, I would increase the sertraline from 50 mg to 100 mg."
C. "Switch from sertraline to fluoxetine if there is no response."
D. "For this patient, I would recommend genetic testing."

6.	Which of the following is true regarding the financing of collaborative care models?

A. Collaborative care codes currently approved by the Centers for Medicare and Medicaid Services allow psychiatrists to bill for time spent in collaborative care activities.
B. There is no evidence that collaborative care for adolescent depression is cost-effective in clinical systems.
C. Consulting psychiatrists who see patients face-to-face for evaluation and treatment planning in collaboration with the primary care pediatrician can bill standard evaluation and management plans for these visits.
D. Value-based payment systems are financially incompatible with most collaborative models.

CHAPTER 49

Collaborating With Inpatient and Subspecialty Pediatrics

Jill Weissberg-Benchell, Ph.D.

1. William is a 16-year-old recently diagnosed with non-Hodgkin's lymphoma. He is actively working with his teachers to modify his homework assignments to accommodate the demands of his chemotherapy. This style of coping is known as which of the following?

   A. Secondary control coping.
   B. Emotional expression coping.
   C. Primary control coping.
   D. Behavioral activation coping.

2. Resilience influences how individuals adapt to a chronic illness and includes which of the following constructs?

   A. Understanding the purpose behind the daily demands of the treatment regimen.
   B. Building skills necessary to promote psychosocial well-being.
   C. Being in the action stage in the stages of change model.
   D. Developing adaptive emotion regulation skills.

3. The consultant and pediatric clinicians are in the same space within the same facility as a team with shared systems and communicate regularly in which of the following models of pediatric consultation-liaison (CL) psychiatry?

   A. Coordinated care model.
   B. Co-located care model.
   C. Integrated care model.
   D. Proactive psychiatric consultation programs model.

113

4. All of the following medications are *not* tightly protein bound except

   A. Sertraline.
   B. Lithium.
   C. Methylphenidate.
   D. Venlafaxine.

5. Which of the following is true regarding the use of psychiatric medications in patients with comorbid epilepsy?

   A. Psychotropic medications are usually not a concern in epilepsy patients because they increase the seizure threshold.
   B. SSRIs, trazodone, and the α-agonists are particularly unsafe to use in patients with comorbid psychiatric illness and epilepsy.
   C. Lithium is considered an anticonvulsant and can always be used safely in epilepsy patients.
   D. Substantial data suggest that stimulants can be used safely, particularly when seizures are well controlled.

PART II

Answer Guide

C H A P T E R   1

Process of Assessment and Diagnosis

Julie Mary Sadhu, M.D.

1. Which of the following is typically *not* a focus of a psychiatric evaluation of a child in the emergency department?

    A. Assessment of risk of harm to self.
    B. Screening for physical abuse.
    C. Planning for appropriate disposition.
    D. Detailed developmental history.

    The correct response is Option D: Detailed developmental history.

    In the emergency department, the clinician will likely be much more directive in the evaluation and will not spend as much time exploring certain aspects of the patient's history, such as developmental history and school history, unless they are immediately relevant to the acute concerns. The focus will be on acute safety concerns (i.e., suicidal risk, homicidal risk, aggression), medical symptoms and conditions, and acute psychiatric issues (e.g., worsening psychosis) and on determining appropriate disposition (whether a child or adolescent requires an inpatient psychiatric level of care, partial hospitalization, intensive outpatient care, outpatient care, an urgent care program, or medical inpatient hospitalization), as well as any need for immediate medication intervention (as in the case of acute aggression or psychosis). Screening for child abuse or neglect is also an important part of an emergency evaluation. **(p. 6)**

2. Which of the following questions would be best for establishing rapport when beginning an outpatient assessment of a 13-year-old adolescent?

A. Why are you here today?
B. What problems do you have that I can help with?
C. How is your relationship with your parents?
D. What grade are you in?

The correct response is Option D: What grade are you in?

For a child and adolescent psychiatrist, it can be helpful to start with an introduction as the "talking doctor" to reassure children that they do not provide shots or physical examinations or procedures and to begin the interview of the child with neutral topics such as age, date of birth, grade in school, favorite subjects (and not-so-favorite subjects), after-school and weekend activities, best friends, sports, and creative activities. This early introductory interview demonstrates to the child and parent that the clinician can talk to kids and collect relevant information and is generally nonthreatening. This allows the child to relax and to view the psychiatrist as a friendly and less threatening individual.

The interviewer can then ask the child what their parents told them about why they were coming to see a doctor today. Asking the chief complaint question this way allows the child to reflect on what the parent told them and avoids putting the child on the spot with such questions as "Why are you here today?" or "What problems do you have that I can help with?" **(p. 7)**

3. When assessing a child's level of functioning during an assessment, what are the five main realms of functioning to consider?

A. Family, peer, school, the child's inner sense of self, and the child's inner world of fantasy.
B. Hobbies, parents, siblings, friends, and pets.
C. School, parents, siblings, friends, and work.
D. School, parents, siblings, friends, and extracurricular activities.

The correct response is Option A: Family, peer, school, the child's inner sense of self, and the child's inner world of fantasy.

Children operate within various spheres or contexts, each of which is significant in their emotional and mental well-being. These *realms of functioning* have been defined as family, peer, school, the child's inner sense of self (including body image and concerns), and the child's inner world of fantasy. Evaluating a child's functioning within each of these realms is a standard part of the assessment. **(p. 4)**

4. Which of the following is *not* a benefit of using standardized rating scales in assessment?

    A. Comparison of the youth with age- and gender-based norms.
    B. Improved diagnostic clarity.
    C. Input from individuals outside the session.
    D. Elimination of the need to interview the parent.

The correct response is Option D: Elimination of the need to interview the parent.

The use of rating scales and forms can assist in information gathering. Using a background questionnaire that asks about family history, developmental history, medical history, and psychiatric history can provide information that will reduce the amount of time required for these topics during the session. The clinician can review this form at the next visit, moving more rapidly through the history sections to confirm and clarify content. Using empirically validated rating scales assists in obtaining a thorough review of symptoms that can supplement the clinical interview, improves diagnostic clarity, and provides information that can be used to further fine-tune the visit, in addition to enabling comparison of the youth with age- and gender-specific norms. The interviewer should focus on domains in which symptoms are prominent and spend more time elaborating on these areas while obtaining at least basic information on other areas. School staff can provide important information about the child's academic functioning, peer interactions, and social and emotional functioning within the school setting. Some parents may not observe or may underreport symptoms that the teacher identifies, and standardized teacher rating scales can be a useful diagnostic tool. **(p. 11)**

5. What is an advantage of the family-based approach to the initial interview?

    A. The adolescent feels more comfortable talking about sexual activity.
    B. The parents and adolescent may have a sense of transparency about the process.
    C. The interview takes longer than the traditional approach of interviewing.
    D. The adolescent is more likely to divulge details about drug use.

The correct response is Option B: The parents and adolescent may have a sense of transparency about the process.

The disadvantages of the traditional approach include the relatively inefficient use of time, increased effort required by the family, and potential delay in treatment. For some families, the clinician's meeting alone with the parent or child may decrease one party's trust in the clinician and even alienate the parent or child, who feels excluded and fears a secret alliance of the other party with the clinician. In addition, individual meetings may risk impairing shared understanding and goals. In some circumstances, time can be wasted repeating portions of the history with each member and/or clarifying or communicating information given by the parent or child.

In the family-based approach, conducting the entire evaluation with both the child or adolescent and the parents in the room, in a way that allows the child to relax with the interviewer and to feel heard, allows the parents to join in and to feel that the interviewer has really understood their child and provides all parties with a sense of transparency about the process and a shared understanding of the presenting issues. However, a potential limitation of this approach is that the interviewer may not feel that the information obtained is complete and accurate if the child or adolescent does not feel comfortable sharing certain items with their parent(s) present. This discomfort may limit disclosure of specific details of sexual activity, substance use, suicidal behavior, or abuse; however, questioning about these topics in the context of the whole family can open up discussion about these concerns. **(pp. 9–10)**

6. McHugh and Slavney's (1998) model for formulation, perspectives of psychiatry, identifies four types of problems common to psychiatry. Which of the following is *not* one of these four types of problems?

    A. Psychiatric diseases.
    B. Disorders related to dimensional or constitutional differences.
    C. Behavioral problems.
    D. Epigenetic factors.

    The correct response is Option D: Epigenetic factors.

    The four types of problems common to psychiatry described in the perspectives of psychiatry formulation model include 1) psychiatric diseases, 2) disorders related to dimensional or constitutional differences, 3) behavioral problems, and 4) life narratives that are problematic to functioning. The *disease* perspective focuses on conditions that affect a patient's functioning (e.g., autism, ADHD). The *dimensional* perspective focuses on extremes in common human characteristics that set up patients to do poorly when there is a mismatch between their characteristic(s) and certain environmental factors (e.g., particular temperaments or personality styles may work in some settings but are vulnerabilities in other settings). The *behavior* perspective emphasizes problems related to choices and activities of the patient (e.g., maladaptive eating and sleeping). The final type of problem, the *life story* perspective, recognizes that the patient's life narrative can have substantial impacts on functioning. Life narratives can range from negative self-fulfilling prophecies to those that empower a person to achieve additional growth (e.g., posttraumatic growth). **(pp. 12–13)**

Reference

McHugh PR, Slavney P: The Perspectives of Psychiatry, 2nd Edition. Baltimore, MD, Johns Hopkins University Press, 1998

C H A P T E R   2

Assessing Infants and Toddlers

Julianna Finelli, M.D.

Mary Margaret Gleason, M.D.

Charles H. Zeanah, M.D.

1. A 3-year-and-4-month-old boy presents with his mother for assessment of dys-regulated emotions and behaviors. The main reason that the caregiving relationship is a focus of the assessment is

    A. The attachment classification determines the diagnosis.
    B. The quality of the caregiving relationship with his mother reflects his other caregiving relationships.
    C. The quality of the caregiving relationship may buffer against environmental risks.
    D. The quality of the caregiving relationship is a good snapshot of this point in time, although it does not have predictive value.

    The correct response is Option C: The quality of the caregiving relationship may buffer against environmental risks.

    Infants who develop a secure attachment relationship with a primary caregiver during the first year of life are more likely to be more resilient in the face of stress or adversity as preschoolers and beyond, have positive relationships with peers, be liked by their teachers, perform better in school, and show more regulated biological stress reactivity patterns. Furthermore, secure attachments buffer stress. In contrast, infants who develop an insecure or disorganized attachment relationship are at risk for a more troublesome trajectory, including early mental health concerns as well as physical health problems.

Attachment classifications may indicate a level of risk, but they do not indicate a specific diagnosis or even the presence of a diagnosable disorder. Children develop unique relationships with each of their caregivers. These relationships are specific, and a child's patterns of behaviors reflect the child's experiences with that caregiver. The quality of the caregiving relationship provides information about the child's experiences with this caregiver up to this point and is predictive of subsequent clinical outcomes. **(pp. 18–19)**

2. A 4-year-and-2-month-old girl is referred to you for evaluation of possible ADHD. Her father is reluctant to attend the first appointment because he thinks she is too young for any diagnostic labels to be considered. You may use which of the following in your conversation with him?

    A. You let him know that DSM-5 includes developmentally specific modifications for all disorders for the preschool age group.
    B. You agree that using diagnostic classifications to describe preschool clinical concerns is a problem because it results in inappropriate "labeling" without clinical value.
    C. You note that insurers will not pay for the care of children's mental health problems, so using a diagnosis is not necessary.
    D. You state that the multiaxial DC:0–5 provides developmentally specific evidence-informed diagnostic criteria to describe clinical mental health concerns in young children and includes a crosswalk to the DSM-5 and ICD-11 systems for billing purposes.

The correct response is Option D. You state that the multiaxial DC:0–5 provides developmentally specific evidence-informed diagnostic criteria to describe clinical mental health concerns in young children and includes a crosswalk to the DSM-5 and ICD-11 systems for billing purposes.

DC:0–5, an empirically derived system of diagnosis for the youngest patients, was published by Zero to Three (2016). This diagnostic approach maintains a multiaxial system that includes explicit attention to the primary caregiving relationship as well as physical health status, developmental status, and caregiving environmental factors.

Although DSM-5 includes more developmental attention than past iterations and includes the first preschool-specific diagnostic criteria for PTSD, developmental adaptations are not available for every diagnosis. Although many people raise concerns about "labeling" a child, it is important to recognize that diagnostic criteria define the child's symptoms, not the child, and precise use of the diagnostic criteria facilitates communication across providers and settings. In general, third-party payers will pay only for care that is deemed medically necessary, which requires a clinical reason for the care, usually in the form of a diagnosis. Although this is not a primary reason for using a diagnostic system, it is a practical factor. **(pp. 19–20)**

3. Which of the following statements is true regarding the comprehensive assessment of infants and toddlers?

    A. Evaluation should begin with focused and close-ended questions regarding the chief complaint.
    B. Only formal, structured observational procedures should be used to assess the parent-child relationship.
    C. Multiple appointments—involving multiple informants and modes of assessment—are typically required.
    D. It is important to conduct interviews and observational assessments of the caregiver and young child individually.

    The correct response is Option C: Multiple appointments—involving multiple informants and modes of assessment—are typically required.

    Assessments of infants and toddlers include multiple appointments, using multiple informants and multiple modes of assessment, including formal and informal observational and history collection procedures. Including the infant or toddler in most appointments can allow for extensive, informal observations of parent-child interactions and reduces the parent's need for childcare during the appointments. As in all psychiatric interviews, open-ended questions are useful. Questions about the child's personality and strengths can be a nonthreatening way to begin the interview. **(p. 23)**

4. The clinician's goal of information gathering in the infant and toddler assessment is to elicit sufficient information to develop a biopsychosocial formulation using all five axes in the DC:0–5. Which of the following is *not* an example of these five axes?

    A. Clinical disorders.
    B. Temperamental traits.
    C. Relational context.
    D. Developmental competence.

    The correct response is Option B: Temperamental traits.

    The five axes in the DC:0–5 are 1) clinical disorders, 2) relational context, 3) physical health context and considerations, 4) psychosocial stressors, and 5) developmental competence. The clinician-parent relationship is central to the assessment and treatment process. Assessment based on this multiaxial system will help the clinician identify the factors affecting a child's emotional and relationship development that will facilitate timely interventions, reduce distress and impairment, and positively influence the child's developmental trajectory. **(pp. 22–23)**

5. A single mother brings her 48-month-old son to the clinic, complaining that he is aggressive and oppositional and has behavior problems at both school and home. The boy is silent and looks at the floor most of the time as his mother talks to the clinician. After obtaining a detailed history of the boy's symptoms, development, social situation, family, and medical history, the clinician wants to assess the boy's attachment to his mother. The most reliable information comes from which of the following?

    A. Themes in the boy's play with and without his mother present.
    B. The amount of protest the boy exhibits when his mother is instructed to leave the room for a brief period.
    C. The degree to which he uses his mother to resolve his distress after the reunion that follows a separation when his mother leaves the room briefly.
    D. The amount of warmth his mother exhibits when describing his problem behavior.

    The correct response is Option C: The degree to which he uses his mother to resolve his distress after the reunion that follows a separation when his mother leaves the room briefly.

    With children whose developmental age is at least 7–9 months, it can be valuable to implement a separation and reunion during the evaluation to provide an indication of how the dyad reconnects following a brief separation. The most important indicator of attachment is the organization of the young child's attachment behaviors (e.g., approach, contact maintenance, avoidance, resistance) *during reunions*. Individual play is not adequate for assessing attachment relationships, and the intensity of separation distress is more reflective of temperamental proneness to distress. The mother's warmth during descriptions of the boy's behavior is useful in assessing their relationship but not sufficient for determining the boy's attachment to her, which requires observation of his behavior. **(pp. 27–28)**

6. In order to assess emotional regulation patterns of a 5-month-old infant with night waking and persistent crying, the clinician would be wise to select which of the following?

    A. The Crowell procedure.
    B. The still-face paradigm.
    C. The Insightfulness Assessment.
    D. Naturalistic observation of parent-infant interaction during history taking.

    The correct response is Option B: The still-face paradigm.

    The still-face paradigm is designed as an assessment of an infant's emotional regulation within a caregiver-child relationship and is appropriate for 5-month-old infants. For infants 3–6 months years old, the still-face paradigm provides valuable information about dyadic emotional regulation. The procedure includes three phases: a naturalistic interaction, a 3-minute period when the parent maintains a nonreactive ("still") facial expression, and a 3-minute reengagement period when the parent interacts as usual.

In the Crowell procedure (Crowell and Feldman 1988), the parent and child (of at least 6 months developmental age) are observed in a series of activities, including free play, cleanup, a bubbles sequence, and four puzzle tasks, as well as separation and reunion.

The Insightfulness Assessment measures a parent's ability to take the infant's perspective and has been used in children from 6 months up to 18 years. In this procedure, the parent is interviewed after reviewing a video of the parent interacting with the child in a structured set of interactions.

Naturalistic observation may provide only limited opportunities to observe dyadic emotional regulation. **(p. 30)**

References

American Psychiatric Association: Diagnostic and Statistical Manual of Mental Disorders, 5th Edition. Arlington, VA, American Psychiatric Association, 2013

Crowell JA, Feldman SS: Mothers' internal models of relationships and children's behavioral and developmental status: a study of mother-child interaction. Child Dev 59(5):1273–1285, 1988 2458891

Zeanah CH, Lieberman A: Relational pathology in early childhood. Infant Ment Health J 37:509–520, 2016

Zero to Three: DC:0–5: Diagnostic Classification of Mental Health and Developmental Disorders of Infancy and Early Childhood. Washington, DC, Zero to Three, 2016

CHAPTER 3

Assessing the Preschool-Age Child

MaryBeth Lake, M.D.

Neha Navsaria, Ph.D.

1. A comprehensive assessment of a preschool child is ideally completed on which of the following schedules?

    A. A 2-hour session, including multiple caregivers and with a brief break.
    B. Multiple sessions on different days with more than one caregiver.
    C. Multiple sessions on different days with the same primary caregiver.
    D. Multiple sessions separated by an hour on the same day with one caregiver.

    The correct response is Option B: Multiple sessions on different days with more than one caregiver.

    A key principle of preschool assessment is that because of significant state- and relationship-related variation in the mental status of the young child, it is necessary to observe the preschooler on more than one occasion and, ideally, with more than one caregiver. Therefore, assessments are best done over a series of several sessions on different days and, whenever possible, with different caregivers. The assessment typically extends over several weeks. Although this is cumbersome to coordinate, changes in the child's behavior, evident within relationships and over time, are invaluable in deriving an accurate diagnosis. **(p. 40)**

2. The format of a preschool assessment based on the Washington University School of Medicine Infant/Preschool Mental Health Clinic assessment paradigm is sequenced with caregivers according to which of the following?

A. Semistructured observation, free play, complete history, review of observations/findings with formulation, differential diagnoses, and treatment plan.
B. Free play, semistructured observation, complete history, review of observations/findings with formulation, differential diagnoses, and treatment plan.
C. Complete history, free play, semistructured observation, review of observations/findings with formulation, differential diagnoses, and treatment plan.
D. Free play, complete history, semistructured observation, review of observations/findings with formulation, differential diagnoses, and treatment plan.

The correct response is Option C: Complete history, free play, semistructured observation, review of observations/findings with formulation, differential diagnoses, and treatment plan.

The format of a preschool assessment based on the Washington University School of Medicine Infant/Preschool Mental Health Clinic assessment paradigm is sequenced in four sessions. Session 1 includes the child's complete emotional, psychological, family, and developmental history obtained from caregivers. Session 2 involves free-play observation with a secondary caregiver. Session 3 includes semistructured observation with the primary caregiver: shared snack, mildly challenging cognitive task, dyadic play, and then separation and reunion. Session 4, with caregivers, includes a review of observations and findings, biopsychosocial formulation, differential diagnosis, and treatment plan. **(p. 41, Table 3–1)**

3. Functional play using objects in ways that demonstrate understanding and exploration of use and function typically occurs at what age?

A. 6–12 months.
B. 12–18 months.
C. 18–30 months.
D. 30 months or older.

The correct response is Option B: 12–18 months.

Observed play in young children can be categorized into the following developmental types: 1) In sensorimotor play I (0–12 months), the child engages in play activity in which the child gains the pleasure of being the cause of action. 2) In sensorimotor play II (6–12 months), the child demonstrates the development of the ability to combine different sensorimotor action patterns into play to explore characteristics of objects. 3) In functional play (12–18 months), the child uses objects to demonstrate understanding and exploration of their use or function. 4) In early symbolic play (18 months and older), the child begins pretend play with increasing complexity and transitions from sensorimotor patterns to mental operations/representations. 5) In complex symbolic play (30 months and older), the child develops play themes with greater imaginative depth, richness, organization, and logical sequence and puts together details of scenes previously demonstrated in isolation. **(p. 43, Table 3–2)**

4. The attunement quality of the caregiver-child dyad refers to which of the following?

    A. Manner and extent to which limits are enforced by a caregiver.
    B. Level of attachment between caregiver and child.
    C. Extent to which the caregiver paces interactions on the basis of the child's signals.
    D. Level of physical or verbal affection expressed toward the child.

    The correct response is Option C: Extent to which the caregiver paces interactions on the basis of the child's signals.

    The attunement quality of the caregiver-child dyad can be understood as the extent to which the caregiver paces interactions in response to the child's behavior, signals, and communication. Questions to be considered in the assessment for evaluating attunement quality include the following: 1) Does the caregiver provide empathic verbalizations or facial expressions? 2) Is there shared joy and excitement? 3) Does the caregiver modulate response to the child's behavior? 4) Is there a pattern of responding *to* rather than *at* the child? **(p. 50, Table 3–3)**

5. Which of the following is the most appropriate cultural interpretation of observed child play during an assessment?

    A. The way in which young children engage with toys is universal and is not influenced by limited access to toys and play opportunities.
    B. Caregivers in collectivistic cultures may engage in one-to-one play less often because of expectations that children are engaged by the extended family/community.
    C. Effects of race and ethnicity are more important than contexts such as poverty and trauma.
    D. Fewer instances of child-directed play signify less parental sensitivity in the parent-child relationship.

    The correct response is Option B: Caregivers in collectivistic cultures may engage in one-to-one play less often because of expectations that children are engaged by the extended family/community.

    A comprehensive evaluation, along with other important aspects, involves a consideration of the cultural context of the preschooler and family. A culturally sensitive model includes an understanding of the child in relation to the family, home, school, community, religion, and society. Collectivistic societies often rely on the extended family or community to engage children in play activities. Such caregivers may appear to place less importance on one-to-one playtime because of their expectation that other adults and children are involved in the child's play.

The way in which young children engage with toys is not universal and is often influenced by limited access to toys and play opportunities.

Culture consists not only of race and ethnicity but also of other cultural contexts, such as poverty, trauma, and the child welfare system. All of these are important to an understanding of culture.

In the cultural aspect of assessment, fewer instances of child-directed play do not necessarily signify less parental sensitivity in the parent-child relationship. Clinicians should engage in the practice of awareness and reflection to prevent judgment and bias from affecting the evaluation outcome and to inform diagnosis and interventions in a culturally competent manner. **(p. 49)**

6. Which of the following represents the typical course of preschool diagnoses of ADHD, oppositional defiant disorder, depression, and anxiety over time?

    A. ADHD persists into school age, but oppositional defiant disorder, depression, and anxiety tend to resolve.
    B. ADHD and oppositional defiant disorder persist into school age, but depression and anxiety tend to resolve.
    C. ADHD, oppositional defiant disorder, and anxiety persist into school age, but depression tends to resolve.
    D. ADHD, oppositional defiant disorder, depression, and anxiety all tend to persist into school age.

The correct response is Option D: ADHD, oppositional defiant disorder, depression, and anxiety all tend to persist into school age.

Longitudinal studies suggest that diagnoses such as ADHD, oppositional defiant disorder, major depressive disorder, and anxiety disorders made during the preschool years persist into school age and therefore warrant early intervention (Bufferd et al. 2012; Finsaas et al. 2018; Keenan and Wakschlag 2002; Lahey et al. 2004; Luby et al. 2014). Early childhood psychopathology also predicts negative social functioning in adolescence. Although studies find that some diagnoses persist beyond preschool age, diagnoses can also change in the preschool and early school period, requiring periodic reassessment (Bunte et al. 2014). **(p. 53)**

References

Bufferd SJ, Dougherty LR, Carlson GA, et al: Psychiatric disorders in preschoolers: continuity from ages 3 to 6. Am J Psychiatry 169(11):1157–1164, 2012 23128922

Bunte TL, Hessen DJ, van der Heijden PG, et al: Stability and change of ODD, CD and ADHD diagnosis in referred preschool children. J Abnorm Child Psychol 42(7):1213–1224, 2014 24781411

Finsaas MC, Bufferd SJ, Dougherty LR, et al: Preschool psychiatric disorders: homotypic and heterotypic continuity through middle childhood and early adolescence. Psychol Med 48(13):2159–2168, 2018 29335030

Keenan K, Wakschlag LS: Can a valid diagnosis of disruptive behavior disorder be made in preschool children? Am J Psychiatry 159(3):351–358, 2002 11869995

Lahey BB, Pelham WE, Loney J, et al: Three-year predictive validity of DSM-IV attention deficit hyperactivity disorder in children diagnosed at 4–6 years of age. Am J Psychiatry 161(11):2014–2020, 2004 15514401

Luby JL, Gaffrey MS, Tillman R, et al: Trajectories of preschool disorders to full DSM depression at school age and early adolescence: continuity of preschool depression. Am J Psychiatry 171(7):768–776, 2014 24700355

CHAPTER 4

Assessing the Elementary School–Age Child

Tareq Yaqub, M.D.

1.   Which of the following is correct regarding interviewing a school-age child?

A. Observations made in the waiting room should not influence assessment.
B. Children often understand why they are presenting to the appointment.
C. It can be helpful to start with normative, nonthreatening questions.
D. Always meet with the parent first to have a better understanding of the child's presentation.

The correct response is Option C: It can be helpful to start with normative, non-threatening questions.

For school-age children, the concept of meeting with a professional to address emotional or behavioral problems may be hard to understand. Initially, asking normative nonthreatening questions is an effective method of placing the child at ease and conveying that their input is important. The observations made while the child is in the waiting room before entering the office can be very important contributors to the assessment. Children can frequently be confused or scared by visiting the doctor and often do not understand why they are presenting to the appointment. Some clinicians prefer to meet with the parent and child together, whereas others prefer to first meet with the parent alone. Although clinicians may use either of these approaches, meeting with the family together helps all feel that their input is equally valued. **(p. 60)**

2. Which of the following is true regarding suicidal thinking and behavior in school-age children?

   A. The child should not be questioned about this directly because it can increase suicidal behavior.
   B. Suicidal thinking and behavior are rarely present in this age group.
   C. Surveys have found a trend toward a gradual decline in suicidal thoughts and behavior over recent years.
   D. Detailed inquiry should be made regarding past and current history of suicidal thinking and behavior, as well as nonsuicidal self-injurious behaviors.

   The correct response is Option D: Detailed inquiry should be made regarding past and current history of suicidal thinking and behavior, as well as nonsuicidal self-injurious behaviors.

   A child should be directly questioned about suicidal thinking and behavior. This approach does not cause the child to be more likely to adopt this thinking and behavior. Far more harm is possible if this line of questioning is excluded. Not only do suicidal thinking and behaviors exist in school-age children, but there has also been an alarming increase in suicide rates in children and adolescents in recent years. Therefore, it is imperative to evaluate for past and current history of suicidal ideation and suicide plans or attempts as well as nonsuicidal self-injurious ideation and behaviors. **(p. 64)**

3. Which of the following is the stage of Erik Erikson's stages of psychosocial development that applies to school-age children?

   A. Autonomy versus shame.
   B. Industry versus inferiority.
   C. Identity versus role confusion.
   D. Trust versus mistrust.

   The correct response is Option B: Industry versus inferiority.

   Erik Erikson (1950) described children ages 5–12 years as meeting the challenge of achieving competence. In this stage, children become much more active in learning and other activities. In most societies, they begin to spend most of their time in school and use learning activities to build a sense of accomplishment. If they fail to make such achievements, children may struggle with inferiority or low self-esteem. Erikson describes this task of achieving competence as the stage of industry versus inferiority, which is the fourth stage of Erikson's psychosocial development sequence. **(p. 66)**

4. Which of the following accurately describes the social development of school-age children?

A. They prefer to interact primarily with their parents.
B. They are not interested in the opinions of their peers.
C. They begin to develop the ability to take the perspective of others.
D. They reject rules and seek out risky behaviors.

The correct response is Option C: They begin to develop the ability to take the perspective of others.

School-age children begin to move away from a world dominated by their caretakers and have an increasing interest in peers and teachers. They are therefore concerned about the opinions of their peers. Children in this period are generally interested in following rules and begin to be able to take the perspective of others. **(p. 66)**

5. Which of the following is the reason that it is often recommended to avoid asking "why" questions to school-age children?

A. Close-ended questions are more conversational.
B. Asking "why" has a higher likelihood of upsetting the child.
C. Responding to "why" questions requires analytical thinking beyond the abilities of most children this age.
D. Asking "why" is not helpful in play therapy.

The correct response is Option C: Responding to "why" questions requires analytical thinking beyond the abilities of most children this age.

School-age children have limited analytic abilities, which makes it difficult for them to answer "why" questions. It is therefore recommended that clinicians use questions that start with "what," "where," or "how." To further facilitate discussion and engagement, it may be helpful to ask questions with reference to recognizable time markers, such as a birthday or vacation. **(p. 67)**

Reference

Erikson EH: Childhood and Society. New York, WW Norton, 1950

CHAPTER 5

Assessing Adolescents

Shirley Alleyne, M.B., B.S.
Steven P. Cuffe, M.D.

1.   Which of the following statements on adolescent psychiatric symptom reporting is correct?

A. Parents report more accurately on internalizing symptoms.
B. Parents and adolescents often disagree on symptom reporting.
C. Adolescents report more accurately on externalizing symptoms.
D. Collateral information from external sources is seldom necessary.

The correct response is Option B: Parents and adolescents often disagree on symptom reporting.

A comprehensive evaluation plan must be developed to accomplish clinically useful adolescent evaluation, including information from multiple sources. Adolescents and parents often do not agree on symptom reporting and have, at best, only modest agreement in their reporting of behaviors and symptoms. More specifically, parents tend to report externalizing symptoms and behaviors more accurately, and adolescents tend to report more accurately on their internalizing symptoms. Information gathering should include collateral information from external sources such as schools and any agencies involved. **(pp. 77–78)**

2.   When resistance occurs in adolescent interviews, what approach should interviewers take?

A. Move to another topic to avoid offending the adolescent.
B. Discontinue the interview to preserve the alliance.
C. Use interviewing techniques to address resistance.
D. Refocus on accessing information from the parents.

The correct response is Option C: Use interviewing techniques to address resistance.

In the initial individual meetings with the adolescent, the interviewer must balance focus on rapport building with data collection. Both need to be accomplished, but excessive focus on one can undermine the other. Moving to another topic, discontinuing the interview, and refocusing on gathering information from parents are not generally helpful strategies. The implementation of various interviewing techniques would address complex issues such as resistance. As an example of resistance, an adolescent may deny having any problems or shrug and say "I don't know" when asked for ideas about problems. The interview engagement process can be conceived of as a cycle that includes the following elements: 1) The clinician engages the adolescent and seeks to understand their concerns, fears, and hopes. 2) The clinician conveys this understanding to the adolescent. 3) The adolescent begins to feel understood and to see the clinician as an ally, leading to the clinician's improved ability to collect accurate data. 4) The clinician uses data collection to increase understanding of the patient's problems. 5) The clinician conveys this increased understanding to improve engagement with the adolescent. **(pp. 80–82)**

3.   Which of the following techniques is used to capture the family history of mental illness in adolescent interviews?

A. Developing a three-generation family genogram.
B. Administering mental health rating scales to family members.
C. Conducting interviews with multiple family members.
D. Reviewing the medical records of family members.

The correct response is Option A: Developing a three-generation family genogram.

A thorough family history of mental disorders should be obtained. A family genogram, which is a diagram of the family history and relationship patterns of three or more generations of family members, is a helpful tool for organizing this information. In addition, if information is obtained during the parent interview that one or both parents have experienced psychiatric or emotional problems, the clinician should strongly consider conducting individual interviews with each parent to further explore how these problems may have affected the adolescent. **(p. 84)**

4.   Why is assessing family structure important to the evaluation of adolescents?

A. It establishes the adolescent's clinical diagnosis.
B. It helps the clinician eliminate potential diagnoses.
C. It establishes the transactional patterns in the family.
D. It determines the clinician's treatment interventions.

The correct response is Option C: It establishes the transactional patterns in the family.

Per Minuchin (1974), family structure refers to the important relationships and boundaries within families and the transactional patterns within these relationships. Boundaries should exist between generational elements in the family, such as between parent and child. Elements of family structure include its ability to change and adapt to new circumstances (adaptability) and the degree of cohesion among the family members. Although the assessment of family structure would help with the process of clinical diagnosis and treatment, it is not sufficient to clearly establish or eliminate a diagnosis and does not determine treatment interventions. **(p. 85)**

5.   Why is it important to assess the adolescent's digital media use during the initial evaluation?

A. It is associated with certain conditions such as autism spectrum disorder.
B. It is associated with improved cognitive functioning.
C. It is associated with better interpersonal relationships.
D. It is associated with worsening mental health.

The correct response is Option D: It is associated with worsening mental health.

Digital media, including any medium that depends on electronics for its distribution (e.g., television, gaming, social media), have become important elements of life in the twenty-first century and are associated with worsening mental health. Although digital media use often leads adolescents to self-diagnose with various conditions, there is no established association with autism spectrum disorder. In addition, there are no studies suggesting improvement in cognitive functioning or better interpersonal relationships with digital media use.

Adolescents, 95% of whom reported having a smartphone according to a recent study (Anderson and Jiang 2018), are often more technologically savvy than their parents and engage in multiple forms of digital media (e.g., gaming, posting to social media websites, texting, live-streaming shows), often simultaneously. More hours spent online are correlated with worsening mental health (Anderson and Jiang 2018). Excessive exposure can be particularly dangerous for youth with preexisting mental illness, those who have low self-esteem, and the socially naïve, making them easy prey for cyber predators. **(p. 76)**

References

Anderson M, Jiang J: Teens, social media and technology 2018. Pew Research Center, May 31, 2018. Available at: www.pewresearch.org/internet/2018/05/31/teens-social-mediatechnology-2018. Accessed July 6, 2020.
Minuchin S: Families and Family Therapy. Cambridge, MA, Harvard University Press, 1974

CHAPTER 6

Neurological Examination, Electroencephalography, Neuroimaging, and Neuropsychological Testing

Sigita Plioplys, M.D.

Miya R. Asato, M.D.

Frank Zelko, Ph.D.

1. Testing with MRI is indicated in which of the following clinical scenarios?

    A. A 15-year-old girl who takes valproic acid for the treatment of bipolar disorder.
    B. A 10-year-old boy with learning disorders and ADHD who often "spaces out" in class.
    C. An 8-year-old boy without significant medical history who developed stereo-typic eye blinking and throat clearing.
    D. A 6-year-old boy with developmental delay and stereotypic episodes of star-ing and chewing behaviors.

The correct response is Option D: A 6-year-old boy with developmental delay and stereotypic episodes of staring and chewing behaviors.

The use of neuroimaging tests to diagnose or suggest treatment for primary pedi-atric psychiatric disorders is unsupported by clinical and scientific data, and there are ethical considerations as well. However, these tests are indicated to rule out neurological disorders with underlying structural, metabolic, or functional brain abnormalities and in research on the underlying neurobiological factors of psychiatric disorders. **(p. 100)**

2.   Which brain waves are present during only the awake state?

A. Delta (1–3/second).
B. Theta (4–7/second).
C. Alpha (8–12/second).
D. Beta (13–20/second).

The correct response is Option C: Alpha (8–12/second).

Typical brain rhythms are classified according to their frequency. Delta waves can be seen in deeper stages of sleep and in pathological states such as encephalopathy. Theta waves can be seen during awake states, although they are more common in drowsy states. Alpha is the predominant wave pattern while one is awake with the eyes closed. Beta waves can be seen during sleep and in patients receiving medications such as benzodiazepines. **(p. 95)**

3.   When there is a clinical need for neuroimaging, which of the following neuroimaging tests is the usual first choice for children and adolescents?

A. Computed tomography (CT).
B. Magnetic resonance spectroscopy (MRS).
C. Functional magnetic resonance imaging (fMRI).
D. Magnetic resonance imaging (MRI).

The correct response is Option D: Magnetic resonance imaging (MRI).

MRI has an extremely good safety profile and does not expose patients to radiation. Thus, it is the first choice for neuroimaging testing in the pediatric population when there is a clinical need. CT is used mainly to evaluate CNS trauma, acute brain hemorrhage, or increased intracranial pressure or when MRI is not available or is contraindicated. MRS provides information on biochemical brain functions and is used to assess metabolic, mitochondrial, and neurodegenerative disorders; to identify an epileptic focus; and in preoperative evaluation of brain tumors. fMRI measures brain energy use during cognitive, sensory, and motor tasks and is most commonly used for preoperative evaluation of hemispheric language dominance for patients with epilepsy and for surgical planning. **(pp. 97–100)**

4.   Which of the following has the weakest indication for neuropsychological testing?

A. To establish a clinical diagnosis of ADHD.
B. To resolve a question of whether a patient has intellectual disability.
C. To evaluate the cognitive basis of functional complaints.
D. To document changes in cognitive functioning over time.

The correct response is Option A: To establish a clinical diagnosis of ADHD.

Neuropsychological evaluation results do not offer incremental utility above and beyond a thorough interview and other clinical information sources (such as parent and teacher rating scales) in establishing a diagnosis of ADHD.

The following are indications for neuropsychological testing: 1) to resolve whether intellectual disability is present, 2) to clarify reasons for lack of response to an educational or therapeutic intervention, 3) to identify areas of cognitive dysfunction that may be related to a medical or neurological disorder, including localized structural or physiological abnormality, 4) to determine the functional significance of a known brain abnormality, 5) to examine the cognitive basis of functional complaints (e.g., poor memory), 6) to evaluate deterioration of cognitive functioning or to document changes in functioning over time, and 7) to assess the prognosis for deterioration or improvement in functioning in relation to treatment (e.g., epilepsy surgery).

The following are contraindications for neuropsychological testing: 1) The patient is acutely ill and mental status is unstable. 2) Uncontrolled (but treatable) ADHD or other psychiatric disorder is present. 3) The patient is in the middle of a medication change with potential cognitive effects. 4) Similar evaluation has recently been completed or is in process (e.g., at school). **(pp. 100–102)**

5.   Which pattern of neuropsychological test results is common to several neurological, psychiatric, and general medical disorders?

A. Disruptions of attention, processing speed, and executive skills.
B. Disruptions of expressive/receptive language skills.
C. Lateralized sensory-motor dysfunction.
D. Significant intellectual disability.

The correct response is Option A: Disruptions of attention, processing speed, and executive skills.

Neuropsychological testing is used to characterize in detail a patient's cognitive functioning compared with same-age peers. In the analysis of neuropsychological testing results, subcomponents of intellectual ability such as verbal comprehension, perceptual organization, working memory, and processing speed are considered in relation to other domains of cognitive functioning such as receptive and expressive language, visuographic and visuoconstructional ability, verbal and visual memory, attention, executive skills, fine motor dexterity, and academic achievement. The focus of interpretation in a neuropsychological evaluation report is the patient's profile of strengths and weaknesses in these domains. Although this profile may be useful in the localization of cerebral dysfunction, it rarely has diagnostic specificity. For example, disruptions of attention, processing speed, and executive skills are common to several neurological, psychiatric, and general medical disorders. **(pp. 100–101)**

6. Which of the following would describe the most appropriate use of neuropsychological testing?

A. A 12-year-old girl with persistent postconcussion symptoms who had previous neuropsychological testing at age 8 years.
B. A 7-year-old boy who is undergoing an individualized education program evaluation at school for a learning problem.
C. A 15-year-old girl admitted to an inpatient psychiatric unit for active hallucinations.
D. A 10-year-old boy diagnosed with epilepsy who had previous neuropsychological testing 3 months ago.

The correct response is Option A: A 12-year-old girl with persistent postconcussion symptoms who had previous neuropsychological testing at age 8 years.

Neuropsychological testing is indicated to identify the cognitive basis of functional complaints such as persistent symptoms following a concussion. The time interval since prior neuropsychological testing at age 8 years is long enough that retesting at this time is not likely to compromise validity due to practice effects. Concurrent testing, such as an individualized education program evaluation at school, is a contraindication for neuropsychological testing. Acute illness associated with mental status changes such as hallucinations is a contraindication for neuropsychological testing. Neuropsychological testing only 3 months after a prior evaluation is contraindicated because of the risk of compromised validity due to practice effects. **(p. 102)**

CHAPTER 7

Intellectual Disability

Parna Prajapati, M.D., M.P.H.

Cheryl S. Al-Mateen, M.D.

Karen Toth, Ph.D.

1. Which of the following would a prudent psychiatrist managing an acute exacerbation of severe irritability and behavior change in an 11-year-old nonverbal girl with severe intellectual disability do first?

    A. Administer risperidone because it is very effective.
    B. Support the caregivers in addressing their burnout.
    C. Rule out nonpsychiatric causes of her presentation.
    D. Administer her home medications because she might have missed a dose.

    The correct response is Option C: Rule out nonpsychiatric causes of her presentation.

    Difficulty in early detection and management of common ailments in patients with intellectual disability who have limited cognitive and communication skills is common. Medical concerns such as urinary tract infections, abdominal discomfort or pain, constipation, or dental pain often go undetected if due diligence is not paid to them during the patient's acute presentations. It is extremely critical to identify and effectively treat the etiology of a sudden change in baseline functioning, which is different from a gradual decline.

    Risperidone is FDA approved for the treatment of irritability in pediatric patients with autism spectrum disorder. However, although it has a strong evidence base in managing self-injurious behaviors and aggression in this population, risperidone is not the next best step because other causes of the patient's presentation need to be ruled out.

Although caregiver burnout is commonly associated with the care of patients with moderate to severe intellectual disabilities, in this patient's acute destabilization, the next best step is to investigate the etiology of this presentation by ruling out medical issues.

Without knowing if the patient is taking any medications or has missed any doses of home medication(s), giving a dose of medication would not be prudent without further investigation. **(p. 124)**

2. A 16-year-old boy with severe intellectual disability is brought to his pediatrician's office for a routine checkup. The physical examination during this visit reveals multiple bite marks on both of his hands and a bald patch of scalp in the occipital region. On further inquiry, the parents report that most of the day he seemed to be in a good mood. They express concerns, however, over the patient's long-standing history of self-injurious behaviors (SIBs) of biting his hands and head banging that have not responded to 3 years of treatment with Applied Behavioral Analysis (ABA). A referral to a child psychiatrist is made at the conclusion of the visit. What pharmacological agent will the psychiatrist most likely consider in addressing the patient's self-injurious behaviors?

   A. Fluoxetine.
   B. Aripiprazole.
   C. Methylphenidate.
   D. No prescription, but a wait-and-watch approach.

The correct response is Option B: Aripiprazole.

SIBs are frequently seen in patients with moderate to severe intellectual disability. Although ABA therapy aims to address these behaviors, it is essential to use pharmacological intervention for those who do not respond to psychotherapeutic interventions. This patient has been in ABA therapy for the past 3 years with no improvement in his SIBs. Hence, the psychiatrist would most likely consider starting a second-generation antipsychotic agent.

The parents report that the patient's mood state is at baseline without significant decline. Therefore, starting an antidepressant medication such as fluoxetine is not the next best step.

Although multiple randomized, double-blind, placebo-controlled studies provide evidence that stimulants may benefit patients with intellectual disability, in this patient's case, no information is provided showing difficulty with attention, distractibility, or hyperactivity, and therefore a stimulant medication is not the next best step.

This patient has not responded to the psychotherapeutic interventions that have been in place for the past 3 years; hence, the wait-and-watch approach with only therapeutic interventions is unlikely to change the concerning behaviors. **(pp. 126–128)**

3. An evidence-based assessment for establishing a diagnosis of intellectual disability must include which of the following?

    A. Standardized intelligence test scores, adaptive assessment completed by a caregiver, genetic testing, and neurological assessment.
    B. Behavioral observations, adaptive assessment completed by a caregiver, sensory-motor assessment, and assessment of SIBs.
    C. Standardized intelligence test scores, behavioral observations, adaptive assessment completed by a caregiver, thorough physical examination, and clinical interview.
    D. Genetic testing, thorough physical examination, neurological assessment, and assessment of SIBs.

    The correct response is Option C: Standardized intelligence test scores, behavioral observations, adaptive assessment completed by a caregiver, thorough physical examination, and clinical interview.

    Although a diagnosis of intellectual disability typically involves an integrative approach that includes providers from multiple disciplines, the minimum required for establishing a diagnosis and treatment plan is cognitive, behavioral, and adaptive testing; a physical examination; and a clinical interview regarding developmental and family history.

    Genetic testing and neurological evaluation are often included in the next steps after a diagnosis of intellectual disability has been established but are not required for the diagnosis. However, these additional steps are often important in constructing a comprehensive treatment plan.

    Assessment of sensory-motor functions and any SIBs will often be included in the next steps after a diagnosis of intellectual disability has been established but are not required for the diagnosis. **(pp. 108–112)**

4. The following treatments are evidence-based approaches for treating children with intellectual disability except for

    A. Cognitive behavioral therapy (CBT).
    B. Behavioral therapy (e.g., ABA therapy).
    C. Social skills therapy.
    D. Pharmacological treatment as the sole intervention.

    The correct response is Option D: Pharmacological treatment as the sole intervention.

    Although many children with intellectual disability benefit from medications, integrative, multimodal treatment is essential. Treatment approaches with the greatest empirical support include CBT (individual more effective than group), ABA therapy, pharmacological treatment, social skills therapy, and parenting programs such as Stepping Stones Triple P. **(pp. 124–126)**

5.   Which of the following statements is true regarding treatment outcomes for pa-
     tients with intellectual disability?

     A. Comorbid ADHD can significantly improve response to treatment.
     B. The developmental course and prognosis of intellectual disability remain the
        same regardless of the cause of the disorder.
     C. Patients with Down syndrome show slowed development after age 11 years,
        whereas patients with fragile X syndrome often demonstrate accelerated de-
        velopment after age 11 years.
     D. With appropriate treatments, some individuals gain in adaptive functioning
        and may no longer meet the criteria for a diagnosis of intellectual disability.

     **The correct response is Option D: With appropriate treatments, some individ-
     uals gain in adaptive functioning and may no longer meet the criteria for a di-
     agnosis of intellectual disability.**

     Some individuals can show remarkable improvement with optimal treatment in-
     terventions, to the extent that they no longer meet the criteria for intellectual dis-
     ability. Comorbid ADHD or autism spectrum disorder can significantly impede
     response to treatment interventions. Unaddressed ADHD can lead to barriers to
     learning and can limit the effectiveness of behavioral interventions for intellectual
     disability. Patients with Down syndrome show a significant developmental delay
     between ages 6 and 11 years, and patients with fragile X syndrome demonstrate
     slowed development after ages 9–10 years. **(pp. 122–124)**

CHAPTER 8

Autism Spectrum Disorders

Jennifer Rahman, M.D.

1. Which DSM-5 severity level of classification for autism spectrum disorder would be most appropriate for a child with incomprehensible speech and significant difficulty in all functional domains?

    A. Level 1.
    B. Level 2.
    C. Level 3.
    D. Level 4.

    The correct response is Option C: Level 3.

    According to DSM-5 (American Psychiatric Association 2013), a child with unintelligible speech and global impairments in functioning would best be categorized under Level 3, "Requiring very substantial support."
    Level 1, "Requiring support," would apply if the child can speak in full sentences but with impairment in one or more domains, not in all domains.
    Level 2, "Requiring substantial support," would be appropriate if the child speaks in simple sentences, along with functional impairment in various situations, not global delays.
    Level 4 is not a severity level of classification for autism spectrum disorder in DSM-5 **(p. 138, Table 8–1).**

2. Which of the following is considered a gold standard assessment tool for autism spectrum disorder that combines standardized questions in conversation with semistructured play in activities?

    A. Autism Diagnostic Interview–Revised (ADI-R; Rutter et al. 2013).
    B. Autism Diagnostic Observation Schedule, Second Edition (ADOS-2; Lord et al. 2012).

C. Childhood Autism Rating Scale, Second Edition (CARS-2; Schopler et al. 2010).
D. Modified Checklist for Autism in Toddlers, Revised With Follow-up (M-CHAT-R/F; Robins et al. 2014).

The correct response is Option B: Autism Diagnostic Observation Schedule, Second Edition (ADOS-2).

The ADOS-2 is an assessment tool that takes approximately 40–60 minutes to administer and allows a clinician to observe an individual's communication, social interaction, restricted and repetitive behaviors, and imaginative play skills by incorporating both conversation and semistructured play through standardized questions and activities.

The ADI-R, although also considered another gold standard assessment tool for autism spectrum disorder, is a standardized, semistructured caregiver interview of 93 scripted items assessing individuals with a mental age of 2 years and older, focusing on three functional behavioral domains (restricted/repetitive interests and behaviors, communication and language, and reciprocal social interaction) that usually takes more than 90 minutes to administer.

The M-CHAT-R/F is a two-step parent report tool used for toddlers ages 16–30 months to screen for autism spectrum disorder.

The CARS-2 relies on a clinician's ratings based on observing a child's behavior. **(p. 146)**

3.   Which of the following is a cognitive theory of autism spectrum disorder that refers to the difficulty in thinking from another's perspective?

A. Weak central coherence.
B. Decreased long-range connectivity.
C. Extreme male brain theory.
D. Weak theory of mind.

The correct response is Option D: Weak theory of mind.

Theory of mind refers to the ability to predict someone else's behavior by understanding their perspective or mental state, also referred to as mentalizing.

Weak central coherence can be understood as local, as opposed to global processing bias, resulting in difficulty appreciating the broader context of cause and effect. This is sometimes described as "failing to see the forest for the trees."

Long-range connectivity is an emerging brain finding (not a cognitive theory), informed by studies of school-age children with autism spectrum disorder that suggest that long-range connectivity is decreased, with potential increases in short-range connectivity.

Extreme male brain theory was based on observations that people with autism spectrum disorder tend to score higher on tests of systematization (a pattern common to men) while noting that, in general, women score higher on tests of empathy. **(pp. 142–144)**

4. Which of the following interventions for autism spectrum disorder involves deconstructing target skills and teaching steps in progression until mastery?

    A. Applied Behavioral Analysis (ABA).
    B. Joint Attention, Symbolic Play, Engagement, and Regulation (JASPER).
    C. Picture Exchange Communication System (PECS).
    D. Social Communication, Emotional Regulation, Transactional Support (SCERTS).

    The correct response is Option A: Applied Behavioral Analysis (ABA).

    ABA is based on learning theory and breaks down a goal skill into discrete steps to teach each part in succession until mastery is achieved. It uses rewards to encourage positive behaviors.

    JASPER is a manualized intervention that integrates behavioral and developmental principles to use joint attention, imitation, gestures, and symbolic play to enhance social language skills.

    PECS is an alternative and augmentative type of communication system (which can be implemented via tablet or smartphone) that allows a person to select illustrations to indicate requests.

    SCERTS is a semistructured, manualized educational intervention focusing on interpersonal interactions (to increase positive behaviors and decrease unwanted behaviors) that can be individualized for a child and family to improve communication and social-emotional functioning across various settings. **(pp. 147–149)**

5. Which two medications are FDA approved for reducing symptoms of irritability and agitation in people with autism spectrum disorder?

    A. Fluoxetine and citalopram.
    B. Risperidone and aripiprazole.
    C. Haloperidol and fenfluramine.
    D. Atomoxetine and guanfacine.

    The correct response is Option B: Risperidone and aripiprazole.

    Risperidone and aripiprazole are approved by the FDA for the treatment of "irritability associated with autistic disorder" from age 5 years for risperidone and age 6 years for aripiprazole; both have evidence for reducing symptoms of irritability and agitation such as tantrums, self-injury, and aggression.

    Although the use of haloperidol for the treatment of similar symptoms is supported by some evidence, it has less evidence that is based on rigorously designed studies and is not FDA approved for autism spectrum disorder–related agitation and irritability.

    Fenfluramine, fluoxetine, and citalopram are not FDA approved to treat irritability in autism spectrum disorder. A systematic Cochrane review examining studies of the effects of fenfluramine, fluoxetine, fluvoxamine, and citalopram on clinical global impression scores and obsessive-compulsive and repetitive behaviors in children with autism spectrum disorder found no evidence to support this use of selective serotonin reuptake inhibitors.

Although randomized controlled trials have shown benefits for atomoxetine and extended-release guanfacine in reducing symptoms of hyperactivity in patients with comorbid ADHD and autism spectrum disorder, these two medications are not FDA approved to treat irritability or aggression in autism spectrum disorder. **(p. 150)**

References

American Psychiatric Association: Diagnostic and Statistical Manual of Mental Disorders, 5th Edition. Arlington, VA, American Psychiatric Association, 2013

Lord C, Rutter M, DiLavore PC, et al: Autism Diagnostic Observation Schedule, Second Edition (ADOS-2) Manual (Part I): Modules 1–4. Torrance, CA, Western Psychological Services, 2012

Robins DL, Casagrande K, Barton M, et al: Validation of the Modified Checklist for Autism in Toddlers, Revised With Follow-Up (M-CHAT-R/F). Pediatrics 133(1):37–45, 2014 24366990

Rutter M, Le Couteur A, Lord C: ADI-R: Autism Diagnostic Interview Revised. Los Angeles, CA, Western Psychological Services, 2013

Schopler E, Van Bourgondien M, Wellman G, et al: The Childhood Autism Rating Scale, 2nd Edition (CARS). Los Angeles, CA, Western Psychological Services, 2010

CHAPTER 9

Communication Disorders, Specific Learning Disorder, and Motor Disorder

Moshe Bitterman, M.D.

1. What is the most prevalent DSM-5 communication disorder?

   A. Childhood-onset fluency disorder (stuttering).
   B. Social pragmatic communication disorder.
   C. Specific learning disorder with impairment in reading.
   D. Speech sound disorder.

   The correct response is Option D: Speech sound disorder.

   Speech sound disorder is the most common communication disorder and involves difficulty in correctly and fluently producing speech sounds and word shapes. The difficulty with producing correct speech sounds is persistent; interferes with understandable speech; interferes with effective communication by hindering others from understanding speech; and leads to impaired functioning across academic, work, and social domains. Speech therapy is the treatment of choice; the techniques used depend on the nature of the disorder. **(p. 158)**

2. Which of the following is not a cause of speech sound disorder?

   A. Atypical muscle tone.
   B. Auditory processing disorders.
   C. Delayed phonological knowledge of speech sounds.
   D. Receptive language deficit.

The correct response is Option D: Receptive language deficit.

Causes of speech sound disorder include atypical muscle tone, vocal structure anomalies, auditory processing disorders, lack of phonological knowledge of speech sounds, and speech motor planning deficit. Receptive language deficit is not one of the causes of speech sound disorder. **(p. 158)**

3.   Untreated language disorders increase the risk of which one of the following?

    A. ADHD.
    B. Anxiety disorders.
    C. Self-injury.
    D. Substance use.

The correct response is Option D: Substance use.

A 26-year longitudinal prospective study that compared subjects with speech-language impairment with a matched control group of typically developing youth, starting at age 5, found significantly higher rates of substance use and depression and poorer physical health in those with speech-language impairment (Beitchman et al. 2014). There were no differences in overall psychiatric or anxiety disorder diagnoses between groups. As seen in the multiple outcome measures used over the 26 years, the effects of communication deficits vary according to context and developmental period. On the other hand, the investigators reported that young adults who were diagnosed as children with mild and moderate language deficits and who received early language therapy had mental health outcomes that were comparable to those of the typically developing control participants. **(pp. 162–163)**

4.   Which of the following specific learning disorders is not in DSM-5?

    A. Learning disorder with impairment in mathematics.
    B. Learning disorder with impairment in reading.
    C. Learning disorder with impairment in written expression.
    D. Nonverbal learning disorder.

The correct response is Option D: Nonverbal learning disorder.

Nonverbal learning disorder is a somewhat controversial syndrome that is said to include deficits in processing visual-spatial and nonverbal information, combined with impaired communication and motor skills, resulting in delayed ability to analyze and use nonlinguistic information. It is not a DSM-5 diagnosis (American Psychiatric Association 2013). Sequelae may include impaired academic, emotional, social, and vocational functioning, as well as subsequent behavioral difficulties. Pragmatic language impairment is common. Nonverbal learning disorder is lifelong. **(pp. 168–169)**

5. Which of the following aspects of a specific learning disorder with impairment in reading is not captured by the more commonly used term *dyslexia*?

A. Problems with fluent or accurate word recognition.
B. Problems with reading comprehension.
C. Problems with spelling.
D. Problems with word decoding.

The correct response is Option B: Problems with reading comprehension.

DSM-5 cautions that dyslexia connotes only problems with fluent or accurate word recognition, decoding, and/or spelling. Specific learning disorder with impairment in reading also includes deficits in word reading and reading comprehension, rate, and/or fluency. **(p. 166)**

6. A 5-year-old boy has had difficulty making friends at school, often feeling that people make fun of him. Teachers say that he usually responds appropriately to instructions in class, but he has trouble explaining what is bothering him when distressed. What is the most likely diagnosis?

A. ADHD.
B. Childhood-onset fluency disorder (stuttering).
C. Social (pragmatic) communication disorder (SPCD).
D. Specific language impairment.

The correct response is Option C: Social (pragmatic) communication disorder (SPCD).

SPCD usually manifests between ages 4 and 5 years. Affected children have difficulty using language for social purposes and can make unintended offensive remarks or incorrectly perceive others' remarks as offensive. Criteria for SPCD include difficulty using language for social purposes, problems following rules of conversation, not understanding what other people imply (e.g., in figures of speech, idioms, and humor that depend on context), and inability to adapt communication style to fit the context (American Psychiatric Association 2013). SPCD limits effective communication, social participation, social relationships, and academic and occupational achievement. SPCD is often misdiagnosed as autism spectrum disorder, even when restrictive interests and repetitive behaviors (required for the diagnosis of autism spectrum disorder) are absent. **(pp. 163–164)**

7. A 10-year-old girl with ADHD is noted to have limited vocabulary, poor spelling, and avoidance of written schoolwork. What is the most likely diagnosis, in addition to ADHD?

A. Social pragmatic communication disorder.
B. Specific language impairment.

C. Specific learning disorder with impairment in reading.

D. Specific learning disorder with impairment in written expression.

The correct response is Option D: Specific learning disorder with impairment in written expression.

Specific learning disorder with impairment in written expression often manifests in fourth or fifth grade with delayed oral language, limited vocabulary, sloppy handwriting with poor letter formation, and avoidance of written work. A population-based cohort study found that 57% of girls with ADHD and 65% of boys with ADHD had impaired written expression compared with 9% of girls and 17% of boys without ADHD (Yoshimasu et al. 2011). **(p. 167)**

References

American Psychiatric Association: Diagnostic and Statistical Manual of Mental Disorders, 5th Edition. Arlington, VA, American Psychiatric Association, 2013

Beitchman JH, Brownlie EB, Boa L: Age 31 mental health outcomes of childhood language and speech disorders. J Am Acad Child Adolesc Psychiatry 53(10):1102–1110, 2014 25245354

Yoshimasu K, Barbaresi WJ, Colligan RC, et al: Written-language disorder among children with and without ADHD in a population-based birth cohort. Pediatrics 128(3):e605–e612, 2011 21859915

CHAPTER 10

Attention-Deficit/ Hyperactivity Disorder

Steven R. Pliszka, M.D.

1. Which response best represents the findings of large epidemiological studies regarding the prevalence of the treatment of ADHD?

    A. Nearly 20% of children in the United States are being treated with stimulants at any given time.
    B. Only about 20% of children with ADHD are being treated with medication.
    C. Less than 10% of children with ADHD have received a behavioral treatment for ADHD.
    D. Nearly one-fourth (23%) of children with ADHD have received no treatment at all.

    The correct response is Option D: Nearly one-fourth (23%) of children with ADHD have received no treatment at all.

    For the 2016 National Survey of Children's Health (Danielson et al. 2018), researchers performed telephone interviews of 45,736 parents of children ages 2–17 years. The parents were asked, "Has a doctor or other health care provider ever told you that this child has attention-deficit disorder or attention-deficit/hyperactivity disorder—that is, ADD or ADHD?" On the basis of the responses to this question, the lifetime prevalence of ADHD was estimated to be 9.4%, and 8.4% of the children were reported as having a current diagnosis of ADHD. Of children with currently diagnosed ADHD, almost two-thirds (62.0%) were taking medication, whereas just under half (46.7%) had received behavioral treatment for ADHD in the past year. Of some concern, nearly one-fourth (23.0%) of children and adolescents whose parent reported they have ADHD had received no treatment at all. **(p. 175)**

2. A 10-year-old child presents with a history of inattention and poor grades since first grade. An ADHD rating scale from the teacher places her in the top 95th percentile for inattention symptoms but at the 50th percentile for impulsivity/hyperactivity. The patient also reports depression nearly every day, low self-esteem due to her difficulties in school, low motivation, early morning awakening, and passive suicidal ideation with no history of suicide attempts or self-injurious behavior. This clinical picture is most consistent with which of the following?

   A. Concurrent diagnoses of ADHD and major depressive disorder (MDD).
   B. ADHD with secondary demoralization due to school failure.
   C. Primary MDD misdiagnosed as ADHD in the past.
   D. ADHD and MDD, but stimulant treatment contraindicated because of risk of inducing more suicidal ideation.

   The correct response is Option A: Concurrent diagnoses of ADHD and major depressive disorder (MDD).

   Because treatment of depression rarely leads to remission of ADHD symptoms, it seems unlikely that MDD masquerades as ADHD to any significant degree. If the full DSM-5 (American Psychiatric Association 2013) criteria for MDD are met in a child with ADHD, this most likely represents the full syndrome of MDD and not a state of demoralization due to the ADHD symptoms. The current clinical consensus is that ADHD and MDD represent separate conditions, each requiring its own treatment. There is no evidence that treatment with a stimulant medication increases suicidal ideation. **(p. 176)**

3. Which of the following statements is true regarding the genetics of ADHD?

   A. Mutations in the dopamine transporter show major gene effects and predict response to methylphenidate.
   B. Only 30% of the variance in ADHD symptoms can be attributed to genetics, and the rest is attributable to the environment.
   C. In one study, more than 300 gene variants in 12 different chromosomal locations were related to ADHD risk, indicating that ADHD is a polygenic condition.
   D. Deletions and duplications in the DNA (copy number variants) are principally responsible for the genetic risk of ADHD.

   The correct response is Option C: In one study, more than 300 gene variants in 12 different chromosomal locations were related to ADHD risk, indicating that ADHD is a polygenic condition.

   About 74% of the variance in ADHD traits is attributable to genetics. According to a genome-wide association meta-analysis of 20,183 individuals diagnosed with ADHD and 35,191 control subjects (Demontis et al. 2019), 304 variants surpassing genome-wide significance in 12 independent loci were identified. **(p. 177)**

4.   In neuropsychological testing, in which area are deficits most likely to be found in children with ADHD compared with control subjects?

A. Working memory.
B. Inhibitory control.
C. Sustained attention.
D. Response to reward.

The correct response is Option A: Working memory.

Recent research has suggested multiple cognitive deficits in children with ADHD (Nigg 2005; Sonuga-Barke et al. 2010). Although it is clear that children with ADHD are impulsive behaviorally, it has turned out that inhibitory control, as measured in the laboratory, does not distinguish those with ADHD from control subjects (Lijffijt et al. 2005). In contrast, working memory deficits robustly delineate groups of subjects with ADHD from control subjects, particularly central executive working memory deficits such as updating of working memory, manipulating information in working memory, and mental manipulation of temporal order (Kofler et al. 2018). **(p. 178)**

5.   Which statement best describes the findings of the European ENIGMA-ADHD study with regard to the cortical surface area in a person with ADHD relative to control subjects?

A. No differences relative to control subjects were found in cortical surface area in either adults or children.
B. Smaller cortical surface area was found in frontal, cingulate, and temporal regions, with stronger effects in the child sample.
C. The effect size of the cortical surface area was quite large, approximately 0.6.
D. Smaller cortical surface area relative to control subjects was greater in adults than children.

The correct response is Option B: Smaller cortical surface area was found in frontal, cingulate, and temporal regions, with stronger effects in the child sample.

The European Enhancing Neuroimaging Genetics through Meta-Analysis (ENIGMA) ADHD study of children, adolescents, and adults compared cortical thickness and surface area between control subjects ($N=1{,}934$) and individuals with ADHD ($N=2{,}246$) (Hoogman et al. 2019). This was a cross-sectional design; subjects were not followed longitudinally. In the ADHD sample, cortical surface areas were smaller in children with ADHD, mainly in frontal, cingulate, and temporal regions; the largest effect size was found for total surface area (Cohen's $d=-0.21$). No differences in surface area or thickness were found between ADHD and control subjects in the adolescent or adult groups. **(p. 180)**

6. Which of these treatments for ADHD has *not* been shown to be efficacious in randomized controlled trials?

   A. Methylphenidate.
   B. Behavior therapy.
   C. Electroencephalographic neurofeedback.
   D. Viloxazine.

The correct response is Option C: Electroencephalographic neurofeedback.

Efficacy of electroencephalographic neurofeedback has not been adequately proven in randomized clinical trials.

Stimulant medications such as amphetamine and methylphenidate have shown efficacy in multiple randomized controlled trials.

Recent meta-analyses show that although behavioral treatments may not have a major impact on ADHD symptoms per se (Sonuga-Barke et al. 2013), they can have a more significant effect on comorbid problems such as conduct problems, negative parenting, social skills, and academic performance.

Viloxazine is a norepinephrine reuptake inhibitor with selective serotonin modulation activity that has been used in Europe as an antidepressant for many years. In a 6-week Phase III study, statistically significant improvements in ADHD-Rating Scale-5 total score were observed in subjects treated with viloxazine compared with placebo at week 1 and through week 6 (Nasser et al. 2020). **(pp. 185–189)**

References

American Psychiatric Association: Diagnostic and Statistical Manual of Mental Disorders, 5th Edition. Arlington, VA, American Psychiatric Association, 2013

Danielson ML, Bitsko RH, Ghandour RM, et al: Prevalence of parent-reported ADHD diagnosis and associated treatment among U.S. children and adolescents, 2016. J Clin Child Adolesc Psychol 47(2):199–212, 2018 29363986

Demontis D, Walters RK, Martin J, et al: Discovery of the first genome-wide significant risk loci for attention deficit/hyperactivity disorder. Nat Genet 51(1):63–75, 2019 30478444

Hoogman M, Muetzel R, Guimaraes JP, et al: Brain imaging of the cortex in ADHD: a coordinated analysis of large-scale clinical and population-based samples. Am J Psychiatry 176(7):531–542, 2019 31014101

Kofler MJ, Sarver DE, Harmon SL, et al: Working memory and organizational skills problems in ADHD. J Child Psychol Psychiatry 59(1):57–67, 2018 28714075

Lijffijt M, Kenemans JL, Verbaten MN, et al: A meta-analytic review of stopping performance in attention-deficit/hyperactivity disorder: deficient inhibitory motor control? J Abnorm Psychol 114(2):216–222, 2005 15869352

Nasser A, Liranso T, Adewole T, et al: A Phase III, randomized, placebo-controlled trial to assess the efficacy and safety of once-daily SPN-812 (viloxazine extended-release) in the treatment of attention-deficit/hyperactivity disorder in school-age children. Clin Ther 42(8):1452–1466, 2020 32723670

Nigg JT: Neuropsychologic theory and findings in attention-deficit/hyperactivity disorder: the state of the field and salient challenges for the coming decade. Biol Psychiatry 57(11):1424–1435, 2005 15950017

Sonuga-Barke EJ, Bitsakou P, Thompson M: Beyond the dual pathway model: evidence for the dissociation of timing, inhibitory, and delay-related impairments in attention-deficit/hyperactivity disorder. J Am Acad Child Adolesc Psychiatry 49(4):345–355, 2010 20410727

Sonuga-Barke EJ, Brandeis D, Cortese S et al: Nonpharmacological interventions for ADHD: systematic review and meta-analyses of randomized controlled trials of dietary and psychological treatments. Am J Psychiatry 170(3):275–289, 2013 23360949

CHAPTER 11

Oppositional Defiant Disorder and Conduct Disorder

Christopher R. Thomas, M.D.

1. Which of the following is the central feature of oppositional defiant disorder (ODD)?

   A. Frequent arguments.
   B. Conflict with authority.
   C. Rule breaking.
   D. Irritability.

   The correct response is Option B: Conflict with authority.

   The behaviors characteristic of ODD can lead to difficulties in all realms of social, academic, and occupational functioning. The central feature of ODD is conflict with authority; therefore, problem behaviors are most frequently seen in interactions with authority figures. Requests for or limits on child behavior typically elicit a sharp reaction from the child, and confrontations quickly degenerate into control struggles. The disputes and conflicts may be over seemingly trivial matters, but perceived threats to control and autonomy are critical issues for children with this disorder. Although negative and disobedient behavior can be normative at certain stages of development or in special circumstances, this disorder is characterized by behaviors that are more severe and frequent than normally expected and result in significant functional impairment. **(p. 198)**

2.   Along with ADHD and mood disorders, which of the following is the most relevant comorbid diagnosis for patients with ODD?

A. Autism spectrum disorder.
B. Anxiety disorders.
C. Developmental learning disorders.
D. Intellectual disability.

The correct response is Option B: Anxiety disorders.

The most common comorbid condition found in children with ODD is ADHD, and many children diagnosed with ADHD also have ODD. Another important consideration is the possible presence of an anxiety disorder. Children with ODD appear to be at higher risk for developing an anxiety disorder. Consideration also should be given to mood disorders because antagonistic and disobedient behaviors are often associated features for children with mood disorders, and studies indicate that children with ODD are at increased risk for a comorbid mood disorder. There is no indication of elevated rates of comorbidity for ODD with autism spectrum disorder, developmental learning disorders, and intellectual disability. **(p. 199)**

3.   Which of the following prevention programs has the most extensively tested proven efficacy in reducing disruptive behaviors among at-risk children?

A. The Incredible Years.
B. Nurse-Family Partnership.
C. Families and Schools Together.
D. Reconnecting Youth.

The correct response is Option A: The Incredible Years.

One of the more extensively studied prevention programs for reducing disruptive behaviors among at-risk children is The Incredible Years series, a parent group training approach (Webster-Stratton et al. 2008). There are two versions of this program, one for preschool children (ages 2–6 years) and one for school-age children (ages 5–10 years). Both programs train parents in behavioral management techniques and foster better parenting practices and involvement in their child's education and development. Two additional programs with evidence for preventing oppositional behaviors in at-risk children that use parent group training are the Coping Skills Parenting Program (Cunningham et al. 1995) and the DARE to be You program (Miller-Heyl et al. 1998). **(pp. 201–202)**

4.   On the basis of longitudinal studies, what percentage of youth with a diagnosis of conduct disorder (CD) go on to have antisocial personality disorder as an adult?

A. 20%.
B. 30%.
C. 40%.
D. 50%.

The correct response is Option C: 40%.

About 40% of youth diagnosed with CD go on to have antisocial personality disorder. Even among those who do not, most will manifest significant functional impairment in relationships and work. **(p. 212)**

5.   Which of the following programs is contraindicated in the treatment of youth with conduct disorder?

A. Parent Management Training—The Oregon Model.
B. Multisystemic therapy.
C. Problem-solving skills training.
D. Scared Straight.

The correct response is Option D: Scared Straight.

Certain treatments, such as Scared Straight programs or brief, one-time interventions, not only are ineffective but may exacerbate antisocial behaviors. Two of the most effective treatments for school-age children with CD are parent management training and problem-solving skills training. Two parent management approaches with well-established evidence of efficacy are Parent Management Training—The Oregon Model and group parent behavior therapy. Multisystemic therapy is a treatment for adolescents that is supported by substantial evidence of efficacy in CD. **(p. 215)**

6.   Youth with callous and unemotional traits are more likely to exhibit which of the following behaviors?

A. Sensitivity to punishment.
B. Isolative behaviors.
C. Thrill seeking.
D. Anxiety.

The correct response is Option C: Thrill seeking.

DSM-5 (American Psychiatric Association 2013) introduced the limited prosocial specifier for CD for those individuals exhibiting callous and unemotional interactions across multiple settings and relationships. Youth who meet criteria for this specifier tend to have a more severe form of CD and may not respond to psychotherapy in the same way as others with CD. Youth with callous-unemotional traits are more likely to exhibit fearless and thrill-seeking behaviors and are less likely to have anxiety or sensitivity to punishment. Isolative behaviors are not known to be associated with callous and unemotional traits. Callous-unemotional traits are not unique to CD, and only about one-third of youth with these traits meet criteria for diagnosis of CD. **(p. 207)**

References

American Psychiatric Association: Diagnostic and Statistical Manual of Mental Disorders, 5th Edition. Arlington, VA, American Psychiatric Association, 2013

Cunningham CE, Bremner R, Boyle M: Large group community-based parenting programs for families of preschoolers at risk for disruptive behaviour disorders: utilization, cost effectiveness, and outcome. J Child Psychol Psychiatry 36(7):1141–1159, 1995 8847377

Miller-Heyl J, MacPhee D, Fritz JJ: DARE to be You: a family support, early prevention program. J Prim Prev 18(3):257–285, 1998

Webster-Stratton C, Jamila Reid M, Stoolmiller M: Preventing conduct problems and improving school readiness: evaluation of the Incredible Years teacher and child training programs in high-risk schools. J Child Psychol Psychiatry 49(5):471–488, 2008 18221346

C H A P T E R   1 2

Substance Use Disorders and Addictions

Martha J. Ignaszewski, M.D., FRCPC
Oscar G. Bukstein, M.D., M.P.H.

1. Dr. Smith is a second-year pediatric resident rotating through child and adolescent psychiatry. She is assessing a 13-year-old adolescent girl with a presenting complaint of "overthinking" who meets diagnostic criteria for generalized anxiety disorder. During a thorough review of systems, Dr. Smith learns that the adolescent has used alcohol socially to reduce concerns about negative evaluation by peers and on two occasions has consumed alcohol resulting in blackout and vomiting. The youth's parents are alarmed about the consequences of alcohol use and ask Dr. Smith about the frequency of alcohol use in adolescents. How should she respond?

    A. Dr. Smith should inform the youth's parents that she meets the criteria for a severe alcohol use disorder and that inpatient rehabilitation treatment is indicated.
    B. Dr. Smith should provide education that early adolescence is a period of initiation of substance use, and epidemiological data reveal that adolescents have increasing use of all substances from age 12 through adulthood. Dr. Smith should suggest that further evaluation of the frequency of use and associated negative consequences are needed to guide interventions.
    C. Dr. Smith should normalize adolescent substance use, given that experimentation with substances occurs in this age range.
    D. Dr. Smith should defer this conversation to an addiction specialist because the topic of adolescent substance use is out of her scope of practice.

The correct response is Option B: Dr. Smith should provide education that early adolescence is a period of initiation of substance use, and epidemiological data reveal that adolescents have increasing use of all substances from age 12 through adulthood. Dr. Smith should suggest that further evaluation of the frequency of use and associated negative consequences are needed to guide interventions.

There are two main periods of increasing substance use in adolescence: early adolescence, coinciding with pubertal maturation, and the transition from adolescence to young adulthood. National epidemiological data reveal that starting at age 12 years, adolescents begin using and more frequently use all substances, with use increasing through early adulthood (Degenhardt et al. 2016). The prevalence of adolescent substance use disorder parallels this chronological trajectory.

Further assessment of this adolescent's alcohol use and its social, recreational, and functional impact is needed. In addition, adolescents with mental health conditions should be routinely screened for substance use, given their higher likelihood of risky substance use.

It would be premature to diagnose this youth with an alcohol use disorder or recommend inpatient treatment without further assessment. Brief intervention and positive reinforcement can be beneficial interventions to reduce substance use. For adolescents with diagnosed substance use disorders, less restrictive treatment strategies should be tried first, in addition to psychosocial and pharmacological supports. **(pp. 222–224)**

2. Screening for adolescent substance use is recommended in primary care and emergency department settings and can be performed by using evidence-based screening tools for youth. These may be targeted or universal screens depending on the clinical setting, presenting complaint, and presence of associated risky behaviors. Presence of which of the following suggests that targeted screening, rather than universal screening, may be sufficient because of lack of association with higher risk status?

   A. Mental health treatment.
   B. Forensic or juvenile justice involvement.
   C. Concerns requiring the involvement of child welfare or protective service agencies.
   D. None of the above. Connection with any of the above services is sufficient to require universal screening.

The correct response is Option D: None of the above. Connection with any of the above services is sufficient to require universal screening.

In a primary care setting, questions for all youth about substance use follow a general inquiry about health behaviors and should include questions about cigarette, alcohol, and other substance use, as well as an assessment of associated risky behaviors. In settings such as child welfare, mental health, or juvenile justice, the high-risk status is sufficient to require screening of each adolescent. Screening may be insufficient in adolescents with frequent substance use who have experienced negative consequences following intoxication, and a more thorough evaluation is indicated. **(p. 229)**

3. Many adolescents who use substances have psychiatric comorbidity, including both internalizing and externalizing disorders. Which of the following is best when considering psychostimulant selection for pharmacological management of ADHD in adolescents, especially considering the potential for abuse and diversion?

    A. Dextroamphetamine.
    B. Adderall XR.
    C. Evekeo ODT.
    D. Vyvanse.

    The correct response is Option D: Vyvanse.

    Psychiatric comorbidity is frequent in adolescents with substance use disorders, with prevalence estimates of 64%–88% (Brewer et al. 2017). ADHD is one of the most common concurrent diagnoses in youth in addiction treatment and is over-represented compared with the general population. Suboptimal treatment may be associated with earlier use of substances, more rapid progression to use disorder, and heavier drug use. Therefore, assessment for ADHD and other psychiatric diagnoses is crucial for adolescents enrolled in substance use treatment.

    For the management of ADHD, select treatment options that have a lower risk of diversion or misuse. The use of long-acting or extended-release formulations is strongly recommended. The pharmacokinetic profile of these formulations is designed to work in phases, releasing medication in the morning and throughout the rest of the day, which prolongs the time to maximum plasma concentration and is therefore less reinforcing. Medications such as osmotic-release oral system methylphenidate and lisdexamfetamine (i.e., Vyvanse) may be preferred stimulants. Vyvanse is a pro-drug, and the release of medication is determined by the action to cleave off the amino acid; it has no activity when injected or snorted, and the kinetics prevent the effect of a high dose. Other answer choices do not represent such pharmacological properties.

    Additionally, nonstimulant options should also be explored for individuals with active substance use disorder or those who have a history of diverting or misusing their medication. Medication management for ADHD is associated with reduced symptoms of ADHD and improved executive and psychosocial functioning, but there is a limited effect on substance use. **(pp. 225–226, 235)**

4. Which of the following is not a recommended primary goal of adolescent substance use treatment?

    A. Controlled use.
    B. Abstinence.

C. Harm reduction.
D. Improved psychosocial functioning.

The correct response is Option A: Controlled use.

The primary goal for the treatment of adolescents with substance use disorders is achieving and maintaining abstinence from substance use. Although abstinence should remain the explicit long-term goal for treatment, given the high risk of relapse within 3 months of treatment completion in youth with chronic use, harm reduction may also be an acceptable interim outcome or goal of treatment. Harm reduction represents a spectrum that may include continued use of substances in a safer manner that is associated with fewer adverse events (e.g., reduced rates of overdose and hospitalization), reduced use of substances, and improvement in domains of adolescent functioning. Controlled use of any nonprescribed substance of abuse is not an acceptable explicit goal in the treatment of adolescents. **(p. 232)**

5.   Which of the following is not a first-line medication used to treat adolescent opioid use disorder?

A. Methadone.
B. Suboxone.
C. Hydromorphone.
D. Naltrexone.

The correct response is Option C: Hydromorphone.

The FDA has approved buprenorphine and methadone for the treatment of opioid use disorder in patients ages 16 years and older and naltrexone for those ages 18 years and older. Methadone, suboxone, and naltrexone are a best practice component of treatment for opioid use disorder in adolescents; use for patients younger than 16 years old is considered off-label.

Each medication has a different mechanism of action at the opioid receptor and, therefore, a different risk and benefit profile. Naltrexone is an opioid antagonist and works by blocking the effect of opioids. Naltrexone is also beneficial for relapse prevention in individuals with alcohol use disorder. Suboxone is a medication that combines buprenorphine and naloxone. Buprenorphine works as a partial agonist at the opioid receptor, which makes it well suited to substance use treatment because it has a lower potential for causing opioid-related intoxication and is, therefore, less habit-forming and has fewer side effects than full opioid agonists such as methadone. Naloxone is not active when administered orally and acts as a deterrent for non-oral administration of Suboxone.

The pharmacokinetic profiles of naltrexone and buprenorphine are such that initiation in individuals who are opioid tolerant or opioid dependent needs to occur cautiously and with guidance from experienced clinicians because of the risk of precipitating opioid withdrawal. Methadone, in contrast, is a long-acting full opioid agonist, which can allow for reduced cravings and withdrawal symptoms. All three medications are associated with a reduction in subjective cravings for opioids and limited effect of illicitly used opioids, thereby allowing individuals to develop increased stability. They are associated with reduced opioid use and mortality.

Hydromorphone is a full opioid agonist sold under the name Dilaudid and is an opioid used to treat moderate to severe pain. Similar to all opioids used for analgesia, hydromorphone has the potential to be habit-forming and is not used to treat opioid use disorder. **(pp. 233–235)**

References

Brewer ST, Godley MD, Hulvershorn LA: Treating mental health and substance use disorders in adolescents: what is on the menu? Curr Psychiatry Rep 19(1):5, 2017 28120255

Degenhardt L, Stockings E, Patton G, et al: The increasing global health priority of substance use in young people. Lancet Psychiatry 3(3):251–264, 2016 27993346

CHAPTER 13

Depressive and Disruptive Mood Dysregulation Disorders

Boris Birmaher, M.D.

1.   Which of the following is true regarding major depressive disorder (MDD) in youth?

A. Its symptoms are similar to MDD in adults, but cognitive development of the child and possible difficulties expressing certain symptoms should be considered.
B. It is not usually accompanied by comorbid disorders.
C. It does not last as long as it does in adults.
D. It does not run in families.

The correct response is Option A: Its symptoms are similar to MDD in adults, but cognitive development of the child and possible difficulties expressing certain symptoms should be considered.

Overall, the clinical picture of MDD in children and adolescents is like that in adults. Still, there are some differences that can be attributed to the child's psychosocial developmental stage. For example, when compared with adolescents, children with MDD tend to be more irritable and present with low frustration tolerance, temper tantrums, somatic complaints, hallucinations, and/or social withdrawal instead of verbalizing feelings of depression. Adolescents may also show these symptoms, but they usually have more melancholic symptoms and suicide attempts.

Depending on the setting, source of referral, and method used to ascertain co-morbid disorders, 40%–90% of youth with depressive disorders also have other psychiatric disorders, with up to 50% having two or more comorbid diagnoses (Birmaher et al. 2007). The most frequent comorbid diagnoses are anxiety disorders, followed by disruptive disorders, ADHD, and, in adolescents, substance use disorders.

The median duration of a major depressive episode is about 8 months in clinically referred youth and about 1–2 months in community samples. Although most children and adolescents recover from their first depressive episode, longitudinal studies of both clinical and community samples of depressed youth have shown that the probability of recurrence reaches 20%–60% by 1–2 years after remission and climbs to 70% after 5 years (Birmaher et al. 2007). Recurrences can persist throughout life, and a substantial proportion of children and adolescents with MDD will continue to have MDD episodes as adults.

Multiple studies show that MDD runs in families. In fact, the single most predictive factor associated with the risk of developing MDD is high family loading for this disorder. **(pp. 248, 250–251)**

2. A 15-year-old adolescent with MDD, moderate psychosocial impairment, and family conflicts was treated with supportive and family therapy for 6 weeks with partial response. Which of the following treatments should be offered next?

A. Continue the same psychotherapy until there is a better response.
B. Offer a trial of an antidepressant medication with an appropriate dosage and duration of treatment.
C. Add an omega-3 supplement.
D. Refer the patient to a partial hospitalization program.

The correct response is Option B: Offer a trial of an antidepressant medication with an appropriate dosage and duration of treatment.

Evidence that supportive management may help comes from pharmacotherapy and psychotherapy randomized controlled trials (RCTs), which have shown that up to an average of 50%–60% of children and adolescents with MDD respond to placebo (Bridge et al. 2007). Thus, it is reasonable for a patient with mild or brief depression, mild psychosocial impairment, and the absence of clinically significant suicidality or psychosis to begin treatment with education, support, and case management related to environmental stressors in the family and school. However, if symptom relief is not obtained in 1–2 weeks, more specific psychotherapy and/or medication are required. **(pp. 258–259)**

3.   A 16-year-old female adolescent was successfully treated for an acute episode of MDD with psychotherapy and an antidepressant. To prevent further depressive episodes, which of the following options should the clinician consider?

   A. Continue psychotherapy and the same pharmacological treatment for 6–12 months at the dose that helped the patient.
   B. Discontinue both psychotherapy and medication.
   C. Discontinue psychotherapy and continue with medication only.
   D. Continue psychotherapy but discontinue medication.

   The correct response is Option A: Continue psychotherapy and the same pharmacological treatment for 6–12 months at the dosage that helped the patient.

   The few studies of continuation of pharmacotherapy and psychotherapy suggest that the relapse rate is higher in youth who do not continue treatment, particularly those with residual symptoms (Emslie et al. 2008). Given these data, together with the fact that the rate of relapse is very high even after successful acute treatment, it is recommended that every child and adolescent continue treatment for at least 6–12 months after acute response (Birmaher et al. 2007; Hathaway et al. 2018). Continuation of both psychotherapy and medication treatment is necessary.

   During the continuation phase, patients are typically seen at least monthly, depending on clinical status, functioning, support systems, environmental stressors, motivation for treatment, and comorbid psychiatric or medical disorders. In this phase, psychotherapy consolidates the skills learned during the acute phase; helps patients cope with the psychosocial sequelae of the depression; and addresses the antecedents, contextual factors, environmental stressors, and internal as well as external conflicts that may contribute to a relapse. Moreover, if the patient is taking an antidepressant, follow-up sessions should continue to foster medication adherence, optimize the dosage, and evaluate for the presence of side effects. **(p. 262)**

4.   According to a meta-analysis, the average response to selective serotonin reuptake inhibitors (SSRIs) is 61%, compared with 50% for placebo. Which of the following is *not* true regarding the high placebo response rate with the use of SSRIs for youth with MDD?

   A. Medication dose is not usually a factor in explaining a high placebo response rate.
   B. The inclusion of youth with mild depression leads to a higher placebo response rate.
   C. The high placebo response rate does not correlate with the number of sites for clinical trials.
   D. The presence of comorbid disorders influences the rates of response or remission.

   The correct response is Option A: Medication dose is not usually a factor in explaining a high placebo response rate.

A meta-analysis of all published and unpublished pharmacological RCTs for MDD in youth showed an average response rate of 61% (95% CI 58%–63%) for the SSRI antidepressants and 50% (95% CI 47%–53%) for placebo, yielding a risk difference of 11% (95% CI 7%–15%) (Bridge et al. 2007). From these data, the number needed to treat to yield one response attributable to active treatment was 10 (95% CI 7%–15%). Possible explanations for the lack of difference between medication and placebo include the following: 1) Depressive symptoms in youth may be highly responsive to supportive management. 2) The data included subjects with mild depression. 3) Other methodological issues, such as low medication dosages, may lead to less separation between SSRI and placebo response rates. Interestingly, the separation between the response to SSRIs and placebo was inversely related to the number of sites involved in the study, meaning that a higher number of sites correlates with less separation between the response to SSRI versus placebo. Last, the presence of comorbid disorders does affect the rates of response and remission. **(pp. 259–260)**

5. An adolescent with MDD was treated with an antidepressant, but a few days later, he became more agitated and experienced worsening of suicidal ideation. Which of the following is true regarding the worsening of this adolescent's clinical status?

   A. About 10% of adolescents treated with SSRIs or serotonin-norepinephrine reuptake inhibitors (SNRIs) may develop or experience worsening of suicidal ideation.
   B. Suicidal ideation and suicide attempts are commonly seen in adolescents with MDD. Thus, the suicidal ideation may have existed before the youth started the antidepressant, or it may have worsened before the antidepressant began to exert its effect.
   C. It is a clear case in line with the FDA black box warning that the antidepressants increase or worsen suicidal thoughts.
   D. This may be antidepressant-induced activation that indicates the presence of bipolar disorder.

The correct response is Option B: Suicidal ideation and suicide attempts are commonly seen in adolescents with MDD. Thus, the suicidal ideation may have existed before the youth started the antidepressant, or it may have worsened before the antidepressant began to exert its effect.

In addition to the rare risk of triggering disinhibition or hypomania in certain children, the most serious side effect of antidepressants is the small but statistically significant risk of onset or worsening of suicidal ideation and, more rarely, suicide attempts. However, the increased risk is small; a meta-analysis showed about a 1% risk difference between drug and placebo with respect to suicidal events, with no deaths from suicide (Bridge et al. 2007).

The U.S. adolescent suicide rate declined from the early 1990s to around 2003, coinciding with the introduction of the black box warning on antidepressants with regard to the risk for suicidal events among youth (Olfson et al. 2003). After the black box warning for all antidepressants was imposed by the FDA, the prescription of antidepressants diminished (Libby et al. 2007), and although they were not proven to be due to the reduction of antidepressant use, the rates of youth suicide increased (Hamilton et al. 2007). Over time, the rate of prescription of SSRIs has increased again. However, the adolescent suicide rate has continued to rise, suggesting that factors other than just the rate of antidepressant prescriptions contribute to the suicide rate. **(pp. 260–261)**

6. A 12-year-old girl was treated with the appropriate dose of an antidepressant for an adequate duration but without adequate response. Which of the following is the most appropriate next step?

   A. Stop the antidepressant and start psychotherapy.
   B. Admit her to the hospital.
   C. Combine pharmacotherapy with psychotherapy, preferentially cognitive-behavioral therapy (CBT) for depression.
   D. Add a second-generation antipsychotic.

The correct response is Option C: Combine pharmacotherapy with psychotherapy, preferentially cognitive-behavioral therapy (CBT) for depression.

In a National Institute of Mental Health multicenter study, the Treatment of Resistant Depression in Adolescents (TORDIA; Brent et al. 2008), depressed adolescents who did not respond to an adequate trial with an SSRI were randomly assigned to one of four interventions using a balanced, two-by-two design: switch to another SSRI, switch to venlafaxine, switch to another SSRI plus the addition of CBT, or switch to venlafaxine plus CBT. No differences in outcome were found between switching to another SSRI and venlafaxine, although youth treated with venlafaxine experienced more side effects. However, the combination of CBT plus medication was superior to medication alone. On the basis of this study, for depressed youth who do not respond to an adequate trial of an SSRI, the best next step is to switch to another SSRI and add CBT. This study is one of the few head-to-head comparisons of different antidepressants. Venlafaxine, fluoxetine, and citalopram all had similar response rates. **(pp. 264–265)**

References

Birmaher B, Brent D, Bernet W, et al: Practice parameter for the assessment and treatment of children and adolescents with depressive disorders. J Am Acad Child Adolesc Psychiatry 46(11):1503–1526, 2007 18049300
Brent D, Emslie G, Clarke G, et al: Switching to another SSRI or to venlafaxine with or without cognitive behavioral therapy for adolescents with SSRI-resistant depression: the TORDIA randomized controlled trial. JAMA 299(8):901–913, 2008 18314433
Bridge JA, Iyengar S, Salary CB, et al: Clinical response and risk for reported suicidal ideation and suicide attempts in pediatric antidepressant treatment: a meta-analysis of randomized controlled trials. JAMA 297(15):1683–1696, 2007 17440145

Emslie GJ, Kennard BD, Mayes TL, et al: Fluoxetine versus placebo in preventing relapse of major depression in children and adolescents. Am J Psychiatry 165(4):459–467, 2008 18281410

Hamilton BE, Miniño AM, Martin JA, et al: Annual summary of vital statistics: 2005. Pediatrics 119(2):345–360, 2007 17272625

Hathaway EE, Walkup JT, Strawn JR: Antidepressant treatment duration in pediatric depressive and anxiety disorders: how long is long enough? Curr Probl Pediatr Adolesc Health Care 48(2):31–39, 2018 29337001

Libby AM, Brent DA, Morrato EH, et al: Decline in treatment of pediatric depression after FDA advisory on risk of suicidality with SSRIs. Am J Psychiatry 164(6):884–891, 2007 17541047

Olfson M, Shaffer D, Marcus SC, et al: Relationship between antidepressant medication treatment and suicide in adolescents. Arch Gen Psychiatry 60(10):978–982, 2003 14557142

CHAPTER 14

Bipolar Disorder

Shane Burke, M.D.

1. Which of the following is a required criterion in DSM-5 (American Psychiatric Association 2013) for bipolar II disorder and not for bipolar I disorder?

    A. Episodes are not attributable to the physiological effects of a substance.
    B. Presence of one current or past major depressive episode.
    C. Presence of mood-congruent psychotic features.
    D. Presence of rapid cycling.

    The correct response is Option B: Presence of one current or past major depressive episode.

    Bipolar I and bipolar II disorders are typically differentiated by the presence of a manic or a hypomanic episode, respectively. However, bipolar II disorder also requires the presence of a past or current major depressive episode. Although bipolar I disorder does not have a major depressive episode as a required criterion, at least one depressive episode usually does occur during the course of the illness.

    The specifiers *mood-congruent psychotic features* and *rapid cycling* are possible in both disorders. Criteria for both disorders require that the episodes not be attributable to the physiological effects of a substance. **(pp. 280–286)**

2. DSM-5 criteria for bipolar disorder have evolved over time, and bipolar disorder has subsequently become more narrowly defined. Some children and adolescents who formerly would have been diagnosed with a broadly defined bipolar disorder have been recategorized to the diagnosis of which of the following?

    A. Major depressive disorder.
    B. Dysthymia.
    C. Disruptive mood dysregulation disorder.
    D. Oppositional defiant disorder.

The correct response is Option C: Disruptive mood dysregulation disorder.

DSM-5 introduced the diagnosis of disruptive mood dysregulation disorder (DMDD) to address chronic irritability that exists outside distinct mood episodes. This diagnosis has become a diagnostic home for many children who previously would have been given the broader diagnosis of bipolar disorder.

Narrowly defined or classic bipolar disorder has a highly recurrent course of clearly demarcated episodes with good quality of remission; rapid cycling is rare and may indicate an underlying medical problem such as thyroid disease or dysfunction. Longitudinal epidemiological and high-risk studies suggest that severe mood dysregulation or DMDD in the context of ADHD is not part of the bipolar spectrum, further supporting narrowly defined bipolar disorder criteria instead of the more broadly defined bipolar disorder (Carlson and Klein 2014; Duffy et al. 2020; Pataki and Carlson 2013). **(pp. 287–289)**

3. Research studies suggest that which of the following brain structures has a significant role in bipolar disorder, particularly in the emotional dysregulation aspect of the disorder?

    A. Hippocampus.
    B. Thalamus.
    C. Amygdala.
    D. Basal ganglia.

The correct response is Option C: Amygdala.

Data converge to suggest key roles for the amygdala, the anterior paralimbic cortices, and the connections among these structures in the emotional dysregulation seen in bipolar disorder (Wegbreit et al. 2014). Their widely distributed connection sites suggest that broader system dysfunction could account for the range of functions—from neurovegetative to cognitive—disrupted in the disorder. Studies are limited, however, by small sample sizes and methodological variability. **(p. 291)**

4. Which of the following is a positive prognostic factor in bipolar disorder?

    A. Older age at first symptoms.
    B. Presence of self-injurious behavior.
    C. Comorbidity with ADHD.
    D. Lower socioeconomic status.

The correct response is Option A: Older age at first symptoms.

The best-known longitudinal study, the Course of Bipolar Youth (COBY), included a naturalistic, multisite clinical sample of children and adolescents with bipolar I disorder, bipolar II disorder, and bipolar disorder not otherwise specified (Birmaher et al. 2014). Trajectories of recovery were followed over 8 years. In the group categorized as predominantly euthymic over follow-up, participants were older at the age of first symptoms and less likely to have exhibited self-injurious or suicidal behavior. Overall, their condition was less complicated, with lower rates of comorbid ADHD and anxiety. Rates of psychiatric disorders (bipolar disorder, ADHD, and other disorders) in their parents were lower, socioeconomic status was higher, families were more often intact, and rates of previous physical and sexual abuse were lower. Half of the predominantly euthymic group had no additional mood episodes over the follow-up period compared with the group of participants with more chronic symptoms (49.9% vs. 8.5%). **(p. 293)**

5.   Which of the following is *not* an appropriate intervention for bipolar disorder?

A. Dialectical behavior therapy for adolescents.
B. Psychoeducation to the patient and family about bipolar disorder.
C. Light therapy.
D. Addressing the educational aspects of the disorder through an Individualized Education Program (IEP) or 504 plan.

The correct response is Option C: Light therapy.

Light therapy is not an evidence-based treatment for bipolar disorder. Although medication treatment of bipolar disorder is vital, adequate preparation for treatment is more likely to ensure its success. Six psychosocial interventions are empirically supported for early onset bipolar spectrum disorders: child- and family-focused cognitive-behavioral therapy, multifamily or individual family psychoeducation, family-focused treatment for adolescents, dialectical behavior therapy for adolescents, interpersonal and social rhythm therapy for adolescents, and cognitive-behavioral therapy for bipolar disorders in adolescents. Additionally, providing psychoeducation to the patient and family members about the disorder is critical to successful treatment. Addressing the patient's educational functioning, as appropriate, with teacher rating scales, psychoeducational testing, classroom observation, and development of an IEP or 504 plan supplements other interventions and provides for more comprehensive treatment and greater likelihood of success. **(pp. 297–298)**

6.   A 16-year-old male adolescent is admitted to an inpatient unit because of symptoms that include 7 days of euphoric mood, impulsive behavior, racing thoughts, decreased need for sleep, and pressured speech. He has no past medical history. History is significant for one past major depressive episode. The urine drug screen is negative. Which of the following is an FDA-approved treatment for his current presentation?

A. Aripiprazole.
B. Lamotrigine.
C. Lurasidone.
D. Oxcarbazepine.

The correct response is Option A: Aripiprazole.

The patient is exhibiting symptoms consistent with an acute manic episode seen in bipolar I disorder. FDA-approved treatments for acute mania in adolescents include aripiprazole, asenapine, lithium, olanzapine, and quetiapine. Lamotrigine is FDA approved for maintenance treatment of bipolar disorder in adults; however, it had a negative trial in youth for relapse prevention (Wagner et al. 2006). Lurasidone has an FDA indication for bipolar depression in youth as well as in adults, but it is not approved for use in acute mania. Oxcarbazepine has no FDA indication for acute mania and was not more effective than a placebo in a clinical trial. **(pp. 298–300)**

7.   When considering treatment of bipolar depression in adolescents, which of the following is true?

A. Quetiapine is effective.
B. There is no increase in risk when using a selective serotonin reuptake inhibitor (SSRI).
C. Olanzapine-fluoxetine combination (OFC) is effective.
D. SSRIs are the first-line treatment.

The correct response is Option C: Olanzapine-fluoxetine combination (OFC) is effective.

Three medications (OFC, quetiapine, and lurasidone) have FDA-approved indications for bipolar depression in adults. However, quetiapine was no better than placebo in studies of youth ages 10–17 years (Findling et al. 2014). OFC (response 78.2% vs. placebo 59.2%; Detke et al. 2015) and lurasidone (response 59.5% vs. placebo 36.5%; DelBello et al. 2017) both had positive trials in youth ages 10–17 years.

Antidepressants alone or with mood stabilizers appear to be less useful in children than adults. Moreover, the risk of "switching" or developing mood elevation in response to antidepressant medication is possible, although this is controversial. Activation by SSRIs is more likely in children than adolescents and adults and may occur in 10%–20% of patients. **(p. 301)**

References

American Psychiatric Association: Diagnostic and Statistical Manual of Mental Disorders, 5th Edition. Arlington, VA, American Psychiatric Association, 2013
Birmaher B, Gill MK, Axelson DA, et al: Longitudinal trajectories and associated baseline predictors in youths with bipolar spectrum disorders. Am J Psychiatry 171(9):990–999, 2014 24874203
Carlson GA, Klein DN: How to understand divergent views on bipolar disorder in youth. Annu Rev Clin Psychol 10:529–551, 2014 24387237
DelBello MP, Goldman R, Phillips D, et al: Efficacy and safety of lurasidone in children and adolescents with bipolar I depression: a double-blind, placebo-controlled study. J Am Acad Child Adolesc Psychiatry 56(12):1015–1025, 2017 29173735

Detke HC, DelBello MP, Landry J, et al: Olanzapine/fluoxetine combination in children and adolescents with bipolar I depression: a randomized, double-blind, placebo-controlled trial. J Am Acad Child Adolesc Psychiatry 54(3):217–224, 2015 25721187

Duffy A, Carlson G, Dubicka B, Hillegers MJH: Prepubertal bipolar disorder: origins and current status of the controversy. Int J Bipolar Disord 8(1):18, 2020 32307651

Findling RL, Pathak S, Earley WR: Efficacy and safety of extended-release quetiapine fumarate in youth with bipolar depression: an 8 week, double-blind, placebo-controlled trial. J Child Adolesc Psychopharmacol 24(6):325–335, 2014 24956042

Pataki C, Carlson GA: The comorbidity of ADHD and bipolar disorder: any less confusion? Curr Psychiatry Rep 15(7):372, 2013 23712723

Wagner KD, Kowatch RA, Emslie GJ, et al: A double-blind, randomized, placebo-controlled trial of oxcarbazepine in the treatment of bipolar disorder in children and adolescents. Am J Psychiatry 163(7):1179–1186, 2006 16816222

Wegbreit E, Cushman GK, Puzia ME, et al: Developmental meta-analyses of the functional neural correlates of bipolar disorder. JAMA Psychiatry 71(8):926–935, 2014 25100166

CHAPTER 15

Anxiety Disorders

Jeffrey R. Strawn, M.D.
Tara S. Peris, Ph.D.
John T. Walkup, M.D.

1.   A 9-year-old girl presents to a clinician for an evaluation of increasing anxiety in social situations and avoidance of friends at school. She denies any significant depressive symptoms or symptoms of ADHD. At school, she continues to do well academically but cannot participate in group activities, raise her hand to ask questions in class, or spend the night with friends and describes extreme discomfort in crowds. Her clinician is considering a provisional diagnosis of social anxiety disorder. Which of the following would increase her risk of having an anxiety disorder?

A. Behavioral inhibition.
B. Low levels of family accommodation.
C. The patient's biological sex.
D. A lack of history of early childhood adversity.

The correct response is Option A: Behavioral inhibition.

Behavioral inhibition, the tendency to feel overwhelmed by and withdraw from unfamiliar situations, individuals, or settings, is present in about 15% of children and increases the risk of developing anxiety disorders. Further, this risk is independent of differences in temperament and age. The other options above are not known to affect risk of having an anxiety disorder. **(p. 318)**

2.   A 15-year-old adolescent presents with symptoms of generalized anxiety disorder. He has been working in cognitive-behavioral therapy (CBT) with his therapist weekly for 8 weeks. Which of the following components is associated with

improvement in children and adolescents with anxiety disorders who are treated with CBT?

A. Having a female therapist.
B. Having a gender concordant patient-therapist dyad (e.g., a male therapist with a male patient).
C. More time spent on challenging tasks and exposures.
D. Extensive psychoeducation.

The correct response is Option C: More time spent on challenging tasks and exposures.

CBT for child and adolescent anxiety typically involves multiple components. Among these, exposure practice is crucial for clinical response, and more sessions in which it is practiced and more time spent on challenging tasks predict improvement. There is no evidence to support roles of gender pairing being of any clinical value. Although psychoeducation is important, it is not known to improve anxiety disorder in children and adolescents who are treated with CBT. **(p. 334)**

3. Which class of medications is associated with greater and faster improvement in anxiety symptoms in children and adolescents who have generalized, separation, and/or social anxiety disorders?

A. α_2-Agonists.
B. Benzodiazepines.
C. Serotonin-norepinephrine reuptake inhibitors (SNRIs).
D. Selective serotonin reuptake inhibitors (SSRIs).

The correct response is Option D: Selective serotonin reuptake inhibitors (SSRIs).

SSRIs, SNRIs, tricyclic antidepressants, benzodiazepines, α_2-agonists, and other classes of medication have been systematically evaluated for the treatment of anxiety disorders in children and adolescents. Among these, SSRIs and SNRIs are the most consistently studied and have been demonstrated to be efficacious compared with placebo. Compared with SNRIs, SSRIs produce faster and greater improvement. **(pp. 330–331)**

4. A 10-year-old boy presents with anxiety symptoms that have been increasing over the past 8 months and are not associated with any recent environmental changes or external factors. He worries about his parents, getting into car accidents, becoming ill, and making mistakes. His parents describe him as "self-conscious." He frequently apologizes and worries that he has upset teachers, classmates, and parents. He notes high levels of tension and restlessness, struggles to fall asleep, and has a sleep latency of 90 minutes. His child and adolescent psychiatrist has recommended a combination of psychotherapy and medication and begins him on sertraline 12.5 mg/day. The child and adolescent psychiatrist wishes to track his symptoms over the course of treatment. Which would be the most appropriate instrument?

A. Hamilton Anxiety Rating Scale (HAM-A).
B. Screen for Child Anxiety Related Emotional Disorders (SCARED).
C. Kiddie Schedule for Affective Disorders and Schizophrenia (K-SADS).
D. Anxiety Disorders Interview Schedule (ADIS).

The correct response is Option B: Screen for Child Anxiety Related Emotional Disorders (SCARED).

Multiple rating scales have been developed to screen for anxiety disorders and track pediatric patients' anxiety symptoms. These symptom inventories facilitate screening and the ability to monitor symptoms over time in both clinical practice and clinical research. Importantly, some scales that effectively assess anxiety symptoms in adults are difficult to use in pediatric patients, even though they have been used in some clinical trials with anxious youth. For example, the HAM-A overweights somatic symptoms (e.g., autonomic, genitourinary, cardiovascular, sensory) that are less commonly reported in pediatric patients compared with adults and may not fully assess cognitive aspects of anxiety in youth (Crawley et al. 2014; Hamilton 1959). The K-SADS (Kaufman et al. 1997) and ADIS (Silverman et al. 2001) are standardized interviews used primarily as diagnostic instruments.

The SCARED tool is frequently used to screen for anxiety disorders and assess multiple anxiety symptoms (Birmaher et al. 1997). It has been validated in both clinical and community youth populations and in several cross-cultural studies. This instrument requires approximately 10 minutes to administer, includes 41 items, and assesses symptoms of panic disorder (or significant somatic symptoms), generalized anxiety disorder, social anxiety disorder, separation anxiety, and significant school avoidance. **(pp. 327–328)**

5. When used earlier in adolescence, which of the following substances or medications has been associated with panic-related symptoms later in adolescence?

A. Nicotine.
B. Alcohol.
C. SSRIs.
D. Methylphenidate.

The correct response is Option B: Alcohol.

In a study of adolescents that examined the relationship between alcohol use and panic disorder, prior alcohol use was associated with increased panic-related symptoms later in adolescence. Of note, there is also a complex relationship between cannabis use and the emergence (or maintenance) of anxiety disorders. **(p. 322)**

6. In addition to SSRIs, which of the following medications has had positive studies in pediatric patients with anxiety disorders?

A. Guanfacine extended release.
B. Selegeline (transdermal).

C. Vortioxetine.

D. Alprazolam.

The correct response is Option A: Guanfacine extended release.

Guanfacine was studied in pediatric patients with generalized, separation, and social anxiety disorders and performed better than placebo with regard to Clinical Global Impression–Improvement scores, as rated by the clinician investigator. Selegiline and vortioxetine have been studied in adolescents with major depressive disorder and did not separate from placebo. Additionally, studies of alprazolam in pediatric patients have not produced positive results. **(p. 332)**

7.   Which of the following DSM-5 (American Psychiatric Association 2013) anxiety disorders is typically the first to emerge in children and adolescents?

A. Generalized anxiety disorder.

B. Social anxiety disorder.

C. Panic disorder.

D. Specific phobia.

The correct response is Option D: Specific phobia.

Specific phobia is one of the earliest anxiety disorders to appear, typically emerging around age 6 years. Like other anxiety disorders, specific phobia has high homotypic continuity with other anxiety disorders, including separation, social, and generalized anxiety disorders. Typically, the next anxiety disorder to emerge is separation anxiety disorder, followed by social anxiety disorder and generalized anxiety disorder. Panic disorder typically emerges in late adolescence. **(p. 314)**

References

American Psychiatric Association: Diagnostic and Statistical Manual of Mental Disorders, 5th Edition. Arlington, VA, American Psychiatric Association, 2013

Birmaher B, Khetarpal S, Brent D, et al: The Screen for Child Anxiety Related Emotional Disorders (SCARED): scale construction and psychometric characteristics. J Am Acad Child Adolesc Psychiatry 36(4):545–553, 1997 91000430

Crawley SA, Caporino NE, Birmaher B, et al: Somatic complaints in anxious youth. Child Psychiatry Hum Dev 45(4):398–407, 2014 24129543

Hamilton M: The assessment of anxiety states by rating. Br J Med Psychol 32(1):50–55, 1959 13638508

Kaufman J, Birmaher B, Brent D, et al: Schedule for Affective Disorders and Schizophrenia for School-Age Children-Present and Lifetime Version (K-SADS-PL): initial reliability and validity data. J Am Acad Child Adolesc Psychiatry 36(7):980–938, 1997 9204677

Silverman WK, Saavedra LM, Pina AA: Test-retest reliability of anxiety symptoms and diagnoses with the Anxiety Disorders Interview Schedule for DSM-IV: child and parent versions. J Am Acad Child Adolesc Psychiatry 40(8):937–944, 2001 11501694

CHAPTER 16

Posttraumatic Stress Disorder and Persistent Complex Bereavement Disorder

Judith A. Cohen, M.D.

Anthony P. Mannarino, Ph.D.

1.   Which of the following is true with regard to epidemiology, risk factors, and co-morbidity related to PTSD in children and adolescents?

A. Greater trauma exposure and a previous history of anxiety disorder are risk factors for developing PTSD.
B. PTSD is equally common in female and male children and adolescents, and genotype does not contribute to the risk of developing PTSD.
C. Media viewing does not contribute to increased risk for developing PTSD postdisaster.
D. Psychiatric comorbidity occurs in less than 30% of cases in the presence of pediatric PTSD.

The correct response is Option A: Greater trauma exposure and a previous history of anxiety disorder are risk factors for developing PTSD.

Female youth are more likely than male youth to develop PTSD. Genotype can contribute to the development of PTSD. Postdisaster, greater media viewing, delayed evacuation, and peritraumatic panic symptoms contribute to the risk of developing PTSD. Psychiatric comorbidity (e.g., major depression, anxiety disorders, externalizing disorders) occurs in more than half of children with PTSD. **(pp. 351–352)**

2. Which of the following should be included during the initial clinical evaluation of a child who may have pediatric PTSD?

    A. Assessing the child's trauma exposure and symptoms through the use of multiple informants, clinical interviews, and standardized instrument(s).
    B. Interviewing only the child about their traumatic experiences and symptoms in order to preserve the child's confidentiality and trust.
    C. Not asking directly about trauma exposure or symptoms because the clinician has not yet developed a trusting relationship with the child.
    D. Requiring the child to describe all of the details of their traumatic experience(s) in order to master avoidance.

    The correct response is Option A: Assessing the child's trauma exposure and symptoms through the use of multiple informants, clinical interviews, and standardized instrument(s).

    As with all evaluations, it is important to obtain information from parents or caregivers and often others (e.g., educators, pediatricians, child protective services) to the extent that this is possible. By asking children directly about their traumatic experiences and responses, clinicians validate the importance of these experiences, including for children who have lost trust in others as a result of their trauma experiences. However, the clinician should not ask the child to describe extensive details about trauma experiences during the initial assessment because this can lead to the child becoming overwhelmed with intrusive symptoms before having the skills to manage them. **(pp. 354–355)**

3. For children diagnosed with PTSD who do not have immediate safety concerns or apparent comorbidity, what is the initial treatment of choice?

    A. An evidence-based trauma-focused psychotherapy.
    B. A selective serotonin reuptake inhibitor (SSRI).
    C. Combined treatment with an evidence-based trauma-focused psychotherapy plus an SSRI.
    D. Tailoring pharmacotherapy to address the child's most prominent PTSD symptoms.

    The correct response is Option A: An evidence-based trauma-focused psychotherapy.

    Among the available treatment options for childhood PTSD, more evidence exists for trauma-focused psychotherapy than for pharmacotherapy. Therefore, in most cases, clinicians should provide evidence-based psychotherapy before starting medication unless there is a compelling reason to do otherwise. For example, if the child has an immediate safety concern, serious inability to function, and/or a comorbid condition for which medication is indicated, it would be appropriate to start medication in combination with trauma-focused psychotherapy. **(p. 356)**

4. During an initial evaluation, a 12-year-old boy endorses, and his mother confirms, that he was exposed to domestic violence perpetrated on his mother when he was 6–8 years old. He has significant current behavioral dysregulation. Which of the following would be a reason *not* to refer the patient to trauma-focused cognitive-behavioral therapy (TF-CBT)?

    A. The family's desire to receive behavioral- rather than trauma-focused treatment first.
    B. Presence of significant depressive, anxiety, externalizing behavior, and PTSD symptoms.
    C. A history of early complex interpersonal trauma, significant behavioral problems, and PTSD symptoms.
    D. The mother's statement that she may not be able to participate regularly in her son's treatment because of her work schedule.

    The correct response is Option A: The family's desire to receive behavioral- rather than trauma-focused treatment first.

    It is crucial to match services to each family's needs, settings, accessibility, and acceptability and to incorporate cultural and developmental sensitivity into how treatment recommendations are made. Addressing the family's current needs (e.g., managing acute behavioral dysregulation) may help them become more open to recommendations for trauma-focused treatment in the future if needed. TF-CBT is effective for addressing trauma-related depressive, anxiety, and externalizing symptoms as well as PTSD. TF-CBT is also effective for youth who experience any type of trauma, including early complex trauma, with or without significant behavioral problems. Clinicians should be particularly aware of the diverse clinical presentations associated with trauma exposure, including significant physical and behavioral dysregulation. Although TF-CBT is optimally provided to both youth and their nonoffending parents or caregivers, it can be effectively provided to youth alone if a parent or caregiver is not available to participate. **(p. 357)**

5. According to preliminary evidence, which of the following appears to be an effective approach for children with maladaptive grief responses such as persistent complex bereavement disorder?

    A. Providing integrated trauma- and grief-focused interventions.
    B. Providing support groups for surviving parents with no child intervention.
    C. Providing pharmacotherapy for depressive symptoms of persistent complex bereavement disorder.
    D. Providing rebirthing or holding therapy.

The correct response is Option A: Providing integrated trauma- and grief-focused interventions.

Although more research is needed to validate instruments and the addition of prolonged grief disorder in DSM-5-TR (American Psychiatric Association 2022), preliminary evidence suggests that providing integrated trauma- and grief-focused interventions can effectively address children's maladaptive grief responses. Parents may or may not receive parallel interventions in these models, but to date, there is no evidence that support groups for parents without including affected children can effectively reduce children's maladaptive grief responses. Pharmacotherapy currently has no evidence to support its use in addressing children's maladaptive grief responses. Rebirthing and other unproven techniques that restrict children's movements have sometimes been used for traumatized children; these methods have led to dangerous complications, including death, and should not be used. **(p. 361)**

6. The cognitive-behavioral intervention for trauma in schools (CBITS) has similar components as in TF-CBT. Which of the following is correct when CBITS is compared with TF-CBT?

   A. CBITS is delivered as group therapy.
   B. CBITS ensures parental presence.
   C. Trauma narrative is an important component of TF-CBT but not CBITS.
   D. The acronym PRACTICE summarizes the core components of CBITS: psychoeducation and parenting skills, relaxation, affective modulation, cognitive processing, trauma narration and processing, in vivo mastery of trauma reminders, conjoint child-parent sessions, and enhancing safety.

The correct response is Option A: CBITS is delivered as group therapy.

CBITS has similar components as in TF-CBT, except that CBITS is delivered as group therapy. Because CBITS is usually provided during the school day, parents are not present. The creation of the trauma narrative during CBITS occurs in individual breakout sessions with the group therapist. The core components of TF-CBT, not CBITS, are summarized by the acronym PRACTICE: psychoeducation and parenting skills, relaxation, affective modulation, cognitive processing, trauma narration and processing, in vivo mastery of trauma reminders, conjoint child-parent sessions, and enhancing safety. **(pp. 357–358)**

Reference

American Psychiatric Association: Diagnostic and Statistical Manual of Mental Disorders, 5th Edition, Text Revision. Washington, DC, American Psychiatric Association, 2022

CHAPTER 17

Obsessive-Compulsive Disorder

Daniel A. Geller, M.B.B.S., FRACP
McKenzie Schuyler, B.S.

1. Although DSM-5 (American Psychiatric Association 2013) uses the same diagnostic criteria for OCD affecting children and adolescents as for adults, pediatric-onset OCD is distinct in several important ways, including which of the following?

    A. A distinct pattern of OCD symptoms that follow developmental themes and distinct psychiatric comorbidity.
    B. Lower familial occurrence in first-degree relatives.
    C. An adolescent peak of age at onset.
    D. A poorer prognosis than for adult-onset OCD.

    The correct response is Option A: A distinct pattern of OCD symptoms that follow developmental themes and distinct psychiatric comorbidity.

    Pediatric OCD shows a distinct pattern of OCD symptoms that follow developmental themes and distinct psychiatric comorbidity. Children's obsessions often center on fear of a catastrophic family event or loss (e.g., death of a parent), leading to checking and other behaviors resembling separation anxiety disorder. Religious and sexual obsessions may be overrepresented in adolescents compared with children and adults. Samples of youth with OCD consistently have high rates of not only tic disorders but also mood, anxiety, and disruptive behavior disorders, ADHD, and specific developmental disorders. There is a small but notable

---

This chapter is dedicated to the memory of Henrietta Leonard, M.D., esteemed clinician, researcher, teacher, mentor, and colleague.

overlap with autism spectrum disorder that can create a challenge for differential diagnosis.

Although family studies consistently demonstrate that OCD is familial, the risk of OCD in first-degree relatives appears to be greater for index cases with childhood onset, with age-corrected morbid risks of 24%–26% (do Rosario-Campos et al. 2005).

The mean age at onset of OCD is 9–10 years, with the majority of childhood-onset disorder emerging between ages 6.5 and 12.5 years.

The recent follow-up report of the Nordic Long-Term OCD Treatment Study (NordLOTS; Melin et al. 2020) found that, with an extended treatment protocol that offered stepped evidence-based treatment over a sustained period, 90% of enrolled children with OCD were rated as responders, and 73% were in clinical remission at 3-year follow-up, using an intent-to-treat analysis. These response and remission rates suggest a better prognosis than for adults. **(pp. 367–370, 373)**

2. Involvement of family members in OCD behaviors in youth with OCD, known as *family accommodation*, is common. Which of the following is true regarding addressing family accommodation?

A. It requires disengagement of accommodating family members in order to provide effective cognitive-behavioral therapy (CBT).
B. It will enhance avoidance behaviors that are needed to decrease rituals.
C. It can be quantitatively assessed using a family accommodation scale.
D. It has little impact on treatment outcome.

The correct response is Option C: It can be quantitatively assessed using a family accommodation scale.

The Family Accommodation Scale for OCD–Interviewer Rated (FAS-IR; Calvo-coressi et al. 1999) assesses numerous factors of family involvement, such as time occupied and disruption to family routines as a consequence of accommodation. It is a useful quantitative tool and will show numeric decline with treatment that addresses accommodation.

Engaging the family to educate and address accommodating behavior is important in almost every pediatric case.

Family accommodation often facilitates avoidance and undermines the principles of exposure and response prevention and habituation and consequently can reduce the effectiveness of CBT in decreasing rituals and other obsessions and compulsions. **(p. 373)**

3. Clinical assessment and diagnosis of pediatric OCD are best made in which of the following ways?

    A. Administering the Children's Yale-Brown Obsessive-Compulsive Scale (CY-BOCS; Scahill et al. 1997) to the affected youth.

    B. Using simple age-appropriate probes followed by a more detailed inquiry regarding time occupied by symptoms and the degree of impairment and distress experienced.

    C. After excluding potential differential diagnoses such as autism spectrum disorder and ADHD.

    D. After evaluating for pediatric autoimmune neuropsychiatric disorder associated with streptococcal infections (PANDAS) by clinical inquiry, anti-strep antibody titers, and throat swab where indicated because PANDAS may mimic OCD in youth.

The correct response is Option B: Using simple age-appropriate probes followed by a more detailed inquiry regarding time occupied by symptoms and the degree of impairment and distress experienced.

Simple questions framed in developmentally appropriate language are the first step in assessment. Follow-up questions must assess the amount of time occupied and levels of distress and impairment to determine whether DSM-5 diagnostic threshold criteria are met.

    The CY-BOCS is a "best-estimate" scale that uses information from *all* sources, including youth, parents, and clinicians, to assign scores. By itself, it is not a diagnostic instrument.

    Comorbid disorders are concurrent disorders that represent non-OCD psychopathology and are not exclusionary. A small percentage of youth with OCD will also meet the criteria for autism spectrum disorder, and a higher percentage (up to 25%) have comorbid ADHD.

    PANDAS is often mistakenly considered to be a diagnosis independent of OCD but refers only to the etiology and putative pathophysiology in a subset of affected youth with OCD. **(pp. 373–374)**

4. Which of the following is true about evidence-based treatments for pediatric OCD?

    A. They are less effective for children with severe symptoms at baseline.

    B. They first require adequate management of comorbid illnesses.

    C. They cannot be delivered remotely using telehealth.

    D. They include CBT, pharmacotherapy with a selective serotonin reuptake inhibitor (SSRI), and combined treatment.

The correct response is Option D: They include CBT, pharmacotherapy with a selective serotonin reuptake inhibitor (SSRI), and combined treatment.

Ample evidence from randomized controlled trials (RCTs) supports both CBT and SSRI medication as first-line evidence-based treatments for pediatric OCD. Even children with severe symptoms at baseline can respond very well to evidence-based treatment, and the outcome is generally not affected by baseline severity. The order in which OCD and comorbid illnesses are addressed in treatment depends to some degree on which is most impairing. When mood disorders are present, they may impede successful delivery of CBT and increase the risk of adverse events with medications, such as behavioral activation in youth with bipolar disorder, and require attention first, but this is by no means a rule. Telehealth-delivered CBT has been shown to be superior to placebo in controlled conditions, albeit with smaller effect sizes than in outpatient CBT. **(pp. 376–380)**

5.   Which of the following is true regarding CBT for OCD?

A. It should always be delivered as monotherapy before medicines are introduced.
B. It has the highest documented effect size outcomes when delivered in a rigorous protocol-driven module.
C. It is a form of relaxation therapy employing principles of acceptance and commitment.
D. It can be delivered only by CBT-trained therapists.

The correct response is Option B: It has the highest documented effect size outcomes when delivered in a rigorous protocol-driven module.

Effect sizes of 1 or greater have been reported for high-fidelity CBT, which is considered a very good response. However, conditions such as wait-list controls may inflate the effect size.

There are some circumstances when medication may precede CBT as a first-line intervention or when medications are used concurrently with CBT, and CBT as monotherapy is not a requirement for successful treatment.

CBT employs the principles of exposure and response prevention (ERP). It is designed to lead to fear extinction learning and is not a form of relaxation therapy.

Anyone, including psychiatrists and parents, can usefully employ ERP if the principles are understood. Indeed, daily homework practice of ERP under parental guidance is often prescribed at weekly outpatient visits, with review and troubleshooting of success and failure at these visits. Formal training in CBT can be achieved through mental health education and training programs and behavioral therapy institutes conducted by experts. The main goal is to understand and practice how to apply CBT with fidelity to its ERP principles. **(pp. 376–378)**

6.   Which of the following is true regarding pharmacotherapy for pediatric OCD?

A. It has high rates of serious adverse events and is a last resort in treatment.
B. Pharmacotherapy improves about one-third of children who receive medication.

C. It has modest effects, with typical decreases in CY-BOCS scale scores of 6–8 points compared with placebo.

D. It will show maximum benefits within 8 weeks.

The correct response is Option C: It has modest effects, with typical decreases in CY-BOCS scale scores of 6–8 points compared with placebo.

CY-BOCS scale scores typically decrease by a modest 6–8 points in randomized placebo-controlled trials. SSRIs are typically well tolerated, and 9 out of 10 youth can be successfully treated with these medications. Serious adverse events are uncommon, and FDA black box warnings regarding suicidal ideation or behavior have a number needed to harm of 143. Further, in meta-analytic studies, the risk was confined to youth with depression, and there was no statistically significant risk of suicidal ideation in youth with OCD. Medication as monotherapy or combined with CBT should be considered as a first-line intervention when comorbid depression or other anxiety disorders are concurrent and also in more severe cases because combined treatment results in greater improvement. In RCTs, two-thirds of youth treated with medication improved compared with one-third receiving placebo, with effect sizes between 0.46 and 0.66 (Geller et al. 2003; March et al. 2004). Medication trials typically last a minimum of 12 weeks, but the clinical benefit may accumulate over 6–12 months at a steady dosage. **(pp. 379–381)**

References

American Psychiatric Association: Diagnostic and Statistical Manual of Mental Disorders, 5th Edition. Arlington, VA, American Psychiatric Association, 2013

Calvocoressi L, Mazure CM, Kasl SV, et al: Family accommodation of obsessive-compulsive symptoms: instrument development and assessment of family behavior. J Nerv Ment Dis 187(10):636–642, 1999 10535658

do Rosario-Campos MC, Leckman JF, Curi M, et al: A family study of early onset obsessive-compulsive disorder. Am J Med Genet B Neuropsychiatr Genet 136B(1):92–97, 2005 15892140

Geller DA, Biederman J, Stewart SE, et al: Which SSRI? A meta-analysis of pharmacotherapy trials in pediatric obsessive-compulsive disorder. Am J Psychiatry 160(11):1919–1928, 2003 14594734

March JS, Foa EB, Gammon P, et al: Cognitive-behavior therapy, sertraline, and their combination for children and adolescents with obsessive-compulsive disorder: the Pediatric OCD Treatment Study (POTS) randomized controlled trial. JAMA 292(16):1969–1976, 2004 15507582

Melin K, Skarphedinsson G, Thomsen PH, et al: Treatment gains are sustainable in pediatric obsessive-compulsive disorder: three-year follow-up from the NordLOTS. J Am Acad Child Adolesc Psychiatry 59:244–253, 2020 30768383

Scahill L, Riddle MA, McSwiggin-Hardin M, et al: Children's Yale-Brown Obsessive Compulsive Scale: reliability and validity. J Am Acad Child Adolesc Psychiatry 36(6):844–852, 1997 9183141

CHAPTER 18

Early-Onset Schizophrenia

Anna Sunshine, M.D., Ph.D.

Jack McClellan, M.D.

1. Which of the following environmental risk factors increase the risk of developing schizophrenia?

   A. Prenatal famine exposure and prenatal infection exposure.
   B. Cold and aloof parenting and prenatal famine exposure.
   C. Prenatal infection exposure and cool and aloof parenting.
   D. Living in a rural location and prenatal famine exposure.

   The correct response is Option A: Prenatal famine exposure and prenatal infection exposure.

   Prenatal exposure to famine as a risk factor for schizophrenia is supported by epidemiological studies showing increased rates of schizophrenia among individuals born following episodes of famine. Prenatal infection exposure has also been epidemiologically linked to an increased risk of schizophrenia and is hypothesized to underlie the increased risk of schizophrenia in individuals born in late winter to early spring. Cold and aloof parenting was a previous but now-discredited cause of autism spectrum disorder and schizophrenia. Living in an urban environment, not a rural environment, is a risk factor for schizophrenia. **(p. 391)**

2. Fran is a 16-year-old with a diagnosis of early-onset schizophrenia (EOS) who is presenting to your clinic to establish care. After you review her previous records, which of the following would raise your suspicions for an alternative diagnosis?

   A. Fran does not have any relatives with a schizophrenia diagnosis.
   B. Fran had genetic testing, which revealed a low polygenic risk score for schizophrenia.

C. Fran had an MRI that showed no abnormalities other than slightly lower-than-average intracranial volume.

D. Fran's reported symptoms include hearing voices when she is upset or angry, fraught and intense relationships with peers, and a history of physical abuse and neglect. On mental status examinations, she has been noted to have a linear thought process.

The correct response is Option D: Fran's reported symptoms include hearing voices when she is upset or angry, fraught and intense relationships with peers, and a history of physical abuse and neglect. On mental status examinations, she has been noted to have a linear thought process.

Patients with other psychiatric disorders such as PTSD can present with psychotic-like symptoms, but the symptom reports are usually atypical (e.g., situationally specific hallucinations) and occur in the absence of other characteristic symptoms of schizophrenia (e.g., negative symptoms and thought disorganization). Despite a strong genetic basis for schizophrenia, most individuals with schizophrenia do not have a family member diagnosed with schizophrenia. Neuroanatomic abnormalities are observed more frequently in individuals with schizophrenia, including reductions in the brain and intracranial volumes, but they are not diagnostic. Current polygenic risk scores lack clinical utility for diagnosis or treatment planning because the odds ratios predicting case versus control status are too small. Individuals with EOS often have premorbid histories of learning disorders, motor abnormalities, or other psychiatric diagnoses, including ADHD. **(pp. 390–392)**

3. An 11-year-old girl is brought by her parents to your psychiatry clinic because she has had sudden onset of auditory hallucinations over the past 2 weeks. The parents deny any previous medical or psychiatric concerns and describe a happy, social child who is an average student in school. She is not taking any medications. During the interview, you observe erratic shifts in her mental state and involuntary movements of her mouth and jaw. What is the likely cause of this patient's symptoms?

A. Childhood-onset schizophrenia.

B. Intoxication with older sibling's stimulant medication.

C. Anti-*N*-methyl-D-aspartate (NMDA) receptor encephalitis.

D. Major depressive disorder with psychotic features.

The correct response is Option C: Anti-*N*-methyl-D-aspartate (NMDA) receptor encephalitis.

Anti-NMDA receptor encephalitis is caused by autoantibodies to a subunit of the NMDA glutamate receptor, resulting in fewer NMDA receptors at synapses. Anti-NMDA receptor encephalitis is more common in female patients, is more common in children and young adults, and can be associated with occult cancer (ovarian teratoma). Although patients can present with isolated psychiatric symptoms, presentation in children often includes seizures, abnormal movements, sleep disruption, and autonomic instability. The other options are possible causes of psychotic symptoms in children but are less likely in this case given the rapid onset and association with movement symptoms and fluctuating mental status. **(p. 396)**

4.   EOS differs from adult-onset schizophrenia (AOS) in which of the following aspects?

   A. EOS is diagnosed using different criteria than those used for AOS.
   B. Neuroanatomical changes have been observed only in individuals with EOS.
   C. Individuals with EOS have less severe negative symptoms.
   D. Individuals with EOS are more likely to have premorbid histories of learning problems and/or motor abnormalities.

The correct response is Option D: Individuals with EOS are more likely to have premorbid histories of learning problems and/or motor abnormalities.

EOS and AOS are diagnosed using the same criteria, with the only difference being the age of onset. Neuroanatomical changes, primarily brain volume reductions, have been observed in individuals with both AOS and EOS. Individuals with EOS generally have more severe negative symptoms on presentation and as they age into adulthood than do individuals with AOS. Individuals with EOS are likely to have premorbid learning and motor abnormalities. **(p. 395)**

5.   Which of the following is true about most youth who report hearing voices?

   A. They have schizophrenia.
   B. They have bipolar disorder with psychosis.
   C. They do not have a psychotic disorder.
   D. They will eventually develop schizophrenia.

The correct response is Option C: They do not have a psychotic disorder.

A substantial number of children and adolescents report psychotic-like phenomena. These symptom reports are qualitatively different than true psychotic symptoms, and most youth reporting such experiences do not have a psychotic illness and will never go on to develop a psychotic illness. Reports of psychotic-like symptoms may simply represent misunderstanding the question or developmental expressions of normal psychic phenomena (especially in younger children). Reports of psychotic-like experiences may also be predictive of other types of psychiatric problems (e.g., anxiety, trauma, substance abuse). **(p. 393)**

6.   On the basis of randomized controlled trials (RCTs), which of the following antipsychotic medications has demonstrated the best efficacy for schizophrenia in adolescents?

   A. Ziprasidone.
   B. Risperidone.

C. Asenapine.

D. Long-acting injectables.

The correct response is Option B: Risperidone.

In the second-generation antipsychotic class, risperidone, aripiprazole, lurasidone, olanzapine, and quetiapine are currently FDA approved for the treatment of schizophrenia in adolescents ages 13 years and older; paliperidone is approved for the treatment of schizophrenia in adolescents ages 12 years and older. Randomized controlled trials of ziprasidone (Findling et al. 2013) and asenapine (Findling et al. 2015) have failed to demonstrate efficacy in adolescents with schizophrenia. Long-acting injectable forms of antipsychotics have not been systematically studied in youth. **(p. 402)**

7.   A large RCT that compared risperidone, olanzapine, and molindone for the treatment of EOS found which of the following?

A. Olanzapine and risperidone were superior to molindone in reducing psychotic symptoms.

B. Only 10% of youth continued their initial medication treatment for 52 weeks.

C. There were no differences in weight gain among the three study agents.

D. Molindone was superior to risperidone and olanzapine in reducing psychotic symptoms.

The correct response is Option B: Only 10% of youth continued their initial medication treatment for 52 weeks.

The largest comparative RCT of EOS spectrum disorders compared olanzapine, risperidone, and molindone over 8 weeks and found no significant differences between groups in response rate or degree of symptom improvement (Sikich et al. 2008). When participants were followed for 52 weeks, only 10% had continued taking their initial medication. Olanzapine had a higher risk of weight gain than risperidone and molindone. **(p. 402)**

References

Findling RL, Çavus I, Pappadopulos E, et al: Ziprasidone in adolescents with schizophrenia: results from a placebo-controlled efficacy and long-term open-extension study. J Child Adolesc Psychopharmacol 23(8):531–544, 2013 24111983

Findling RL, Landbloom RP, Mackle M, et al: Safety and efficacy from an 8 week double-blind trial and a 26 week open-label extension of asenapine in adolescents with schizophrenia. J Child Adolesc Psychopharmacol 25(5):384–396, 2015 26091193

Sikich L, Frazier JA, McClellan J, et al: Double-blind comparison of first- and second-generation antipsychotics in early onset schizophrenia and schizoaffective disorder: findings from the Treatment of Early Onset Schizophrenia Spectrum Disorders (TEOSS) study. Am J Psychiatry 165(11):1420–1431, 2008 18794207

CHAPTER 19

Eating and Feeding Disorders

Kamryn T. Eddy, Ph.D.

1. A 15-year-old adolescent presents for an evaluation because of recent weight loss (he has fallen from the 25th to the 5th percentile for BMI). He expresses fear of weight gain and does not understand why his parents are bringing him in for an evaluation. His parents report that they see him eating large amounts of food after school, and they worry that he is making himself vomit. Which diagnosis best fits his presentation?

   A. Anorexia nervosa.
   B. Bulimia nervosa.
   C. Binge eating disorder.
   D. Atypical anorexia nervosa.

   The correct response is Option A: Anorexia nervosa.

   Anorexia nervosa is the best answer because he has lost weight and fallen off his growth curve, leading to low weight (criterion A), expresses fear of weight gain (criterion B), and seems to have difficulty appreciating the seriousness of his condition (criterion C) (American Psychiatric Association 2013). His parents notice behaviors that may suggest binge-eating and purging, which may be consistent with the binge-eating/purging type of anorexia nervosa. **(p. 412, Box 19–1)**

2. The three examples of rationales for food avoidance/restriction in avoidant/restrictive food intake disorder (ARFID) that are described in DSM-5 (American Psychiatric Association 2013) include which of the following?

    A. Lack of interest in eating or food, fear of weight gain, and fear of aversive consequences.
    B. Lack of interest in eating or food, binge eating, and sensory sensitivity.
    C. Sensory sensitivity, fear of aversive consequences, and lack of interest in eating or food.
    D. Sensory sensitivity, fear of weight gain, and lack of interest in eating or food.

    The correct response is Option C: Sensory sensitivity, fear of aversive consequences, and lack of interest in eating or food.

    DSM-5 describes three common rationales for food avoidance/restriction in ARFID, including apparent lack of interest in eating or food, avoidance due to sensory characteristics of food, and fear of aversive consequences (such as choking or vomiting). Symptoms such as fear of weight gain (anorexia nervosa criterion B) and binge eating (criterion A for bulimia nervosa and for binge-eating disorder) do not drive eating behaviors in ARFID. **(p. 415, Box 19–4)**

3. Which of the following is suggested by family-based treatment for children and adolescents with anorexia nervosa and bulimia nervosa?

    A. Dysfunctional family dynamics have contributed to the development of the eating disorder.
    B. Parents must be included in the treatment because they are to blame for causing the eating disorder.
    C. Parents are not to blame for causing the eating disorder and may actually be the child's best resource for achieving recovery.
    D. Parents have very little idea how to refeed their child and typically need help from professionals.

    The correct response is Option C: Parents are not to blame for causing the eating disorder and may actually be the child's best resource for achieving recovery.

    Family-based treatment for eating disorders is agnostic to eating disorder etiology. It views the parents as a resource who can be instrumental in helping the child interrupt symptoms because they are regarded as experts on their own child, have an investment in their child's health and well-being, and (most often) live with their child, giving them daily access for intervention. **(p. 425)**

4. Which of the following is assumed to be the core transdiagnostic mechanism that maintains eating disorders as viewed in cognitive-behavioral therapy for eating disorders?

    A. Dieting.
    B. Binge-eating/purging.
    C. Childhood traumatic experience.
    D. Overvaluation of body weight and shape.

    The correct response is Option D: Overvaluation of body weight and shape.

    Overvaluation of weight and shape, placing great emphasis on the importance of body weight and shape in defining one's self-worth, is considered to be a core maintaining mechanism across eating disorders as viewed in the cognitive-behavioral model of eating disorders. **(p. 428)**

5. Which of the following is true regarding psychopharmacology for eating disorders?

    A. No medications are proven to treat anorexia nervosa.
    B. Fluoxetine is the only FDA-approved medication available for the treatment of avoidant/restrictive food intake disorder.
    C. Medications are not useful in the treatment of comorbidity in individuals with eating disorders.
    D. Olanzapine is the first-line treatment for anorexia nervosa.

    The correct response is Option A: No medications are proven to treat anorexia nervosa.

    Currently, no medications that have been proven to treat anorexia nervosa are available. Understanding the role of psychopharmacology in eating disorders is in its infancy. Although the use of psychopharmacological agents is limited during times of acute medical compromise, low-dose atypical antipsychotics are sometimes used to address associated symptoms such as severe obsessive thinking, anxiety, and psychotic-like thinking. **(p. 429)**

Reference

American Psychiatric Association: Diagnostic and Statistical Manual of Mental Disorders, 5th Edition. Arlington, VA, American Psychiatric Association, 2013

CHAPTER 20

Tic Disorders

Nicole Mavrides, M.D.

Nadina Abdullayeva, M.D.

1.   Which of the following is *false* regarding tics?

   A. Tics are distinguished by urges or sensations that precede the movements or sounds.
   B. Tics follow a specific rhythm and occur regularly in bouts.
   C. Tics may resolve over time.
   D. Complex motor tics can at times appear purposeful, like jumping or kissing.

The correct response is Option B: Tics follow a specific rhythm and occur regularly in bouts.

Tics are sudden, repetitive, nonrhythmic movements in any part of the body or vocalizations that typically wax and wane in frequency and intensity. Tics do not follow a specific rhythm and can occur in irregular time frames over the course of the day, week, month, or year.

   Many patients describe a specific urge or sensation that comes before the expressed movement or sound.

   Tics tend to evolve over time in their severity, complexity, and suppressibility. They also may resolve completely as the patient ages.

   Simple motor tics usually occur from one muscle group—with a twitch or a jerk of facial expressions (blinking) or flexion/extension of the neck, trunk, arms, or legs. Complex motor tics involve more than one muscle group, last longer, and appear more purposeful. Complex tics can involve jumping, kissing, echopraxia (repeating another's motions), or echolalia (repeating another's words). **(pp. 437–438)**

207

2.	All of the following are modifiable risk factors for developing tics *except*

A. Prematurity.
B. Low birth weight.
C. Maternal autoimmune disease.
D. Family history of tics.

The correct response is Option D: Family history of tics.

Family history is the nonmodifiable risk factor for developing tics. Potentially modifiable risks include premature birth, low birth weight, and maternal autoimmune disease. Tics have also been shown to be associated with streptococcal infections, such as pediatric autoimmune neuropsychiatric disorders associated with streptococcal infections (PANDAS). Some additional preventable risk factors include gestational exposure to tobacco, alcohol, and cannabis. Psychosocial stressors can exacerbate tics. **(pp. 440–441)**

3.	Comorbidity with tic disorders and Tourette's disorder is extremely common. Which of these disorders is *not* frequently associated with tics?

A. ADHD.
B. Obsessive-compulsive disorder.
C. Schizophrenia.
D. Autism spectrum disorder.

The correct response is Option C: Schizophrenia.

There is no evidence that patients with schizophrenia frequently have tic disorders or vice versa. Comorbidity with other psychiatric disorders is extremely common, occurring in close to 90% of patients with Tourette's disorder and tics (Coffey 2015; Hirschtritt et al. 2015). The most common disorder seen with Tourette's is ADHD, which increases functional impairment and can be difficult to treat. Although stimulants were initially suspected to worsen tics, they have been shown to improve prognosis in both disorders. OCD can be seen in nearly 50% of patients with Tourette's, and having both disorders can predict a poorer prognosis. Having an early onset of OCD, when peak tic severity occurs, can be associated with resistance to SSRI monotherapy. Some studies have shown that 23% of Tourette's patients also meet the criteria for autism spectrum disorder (Darrow et al. 2017). **(pp. 441–442)**

4.	Which of the following is the most accurate statement regarding the course of tic disorders in an individual?

A. If onset of tics is after age 8 years, the clinician must look elsewhere for the etiology of involuntary movements.
B. Although psychosocial stressors such as teasing may worsen symptoms early on, studies show that these patients develop better coping skills and are more successful and resilient in the future.

C. It is recommended that a person's tics be ignored in all settings; this helps the individual feel included and cared for during the distressing time of tics.

D. Patients with tics or Tourette's disorder have four times the risk of suicide compared with the general population. The increase in risk remains substantial even after adjusting for psychiatric comorbidity.

The correct response is Option D: Patients with tics or Tourette's disorder have four times the risk of suicide compared with the general population. The increase in risk remains substantial even after adjusting for psychiatric comorbidity.

Patients with tic disorder or Tourette's disorder indeed have four times the risk of suicide when compared to the general population (Fernández de la Cruz et al. 2017). The most powerful predictors of suicide in these patients are the persistence of tics beyond young adulthood and a previous suicide attempt.

Tics typically begin in childhood, around age 4–6 years, but according to DSM-5 (American Psychiatric Association 2013), the onset must be before age 18 years; there is no particular clinical relevance to age 8 years.

Predictors of worse outcomes in adulthood include severe tics and being teased in childhood, family history, ADHD, and OCD.

Ignoring tics in all settings can be detrimental and alienating to a child if the child needs reassurance; tics must be addressed on a case-by-case basis. **(pp. 443–444)**

5. Eva, an 11-year-old girl, is brought to your office by her parents for evaluation of tics. As you converse with the parents, you observe both vocal and motor tics in Eva. She also frequently interrupts her parents with her own questions and walks around the office inquiring about posters. She jokes with her father and seems to be enjoying herself. You note that the parents seem uncomfortable with Eva's behavior and are trying to get her to sit quietly. Eva readily understands, apologizes for her behavior, and sits down. Which of the following would be your best next step?

A. Eva's tics are obvious, likely causing significant distress. You should start an FDA-approved treatment immediately to help mitigate the social stigma she might be experiencing at school.

B. Eva is clearly inattentive, intrusive, and hyperactive, and you likely will need to start a stimulant medication to help with her ADHD.

C. You compliment the parents on having such a curious daughter and interview the family further to gather more information about all possible symptoms before prescribing anything.

D. You recommend parent-child interaction therapy because the parents are clearly struggling with controlling their difficult child.

The correct response is Option C: You compliment the parents on having such a curious daughter and interview the family further to gather more information about all possible symptoms before prescribing anything.

Tics are highly variable in presentation and need to be evaluated on an individual basis, carefully assessing their effect on the quality of life of the individual and others. During an initial evaluation, it is important to observe and gather as much history as possible before deciding on a treatment. **(pp. 444–445)**

6. Which of the following is true regarding the pharmacology of tic disorders?

    A. α-Agonists and dopamine blockers have shown equal efficacy in clinical practice, and the choice depends on the family's preference.
    B. The three FDA-approved medications (clonidine, guanfacine, and haloperidol) are the first-line treatment for any type of tics.
    C. Comprehensive Behavioral Intervention for Tics (CBIT) is the first-line recommended treatment for all tics before starting any medication.
    D. Depending on the nature of the tics, effects on quality of life, family resources, and much more, each patient's treatment should be approached on an individual basis, and pharmacology is not always the first step.

The correct response is Option D: Depending on the nature of the tics, effects on quality of life, family resources, and much more, each patient's treatment should be approached on an individual basis, and pharmacology is not always the first step.

Dopamine blockers have demonstrated efficacy but are not generally used as a first-line treatment because of significant side effects. The three medications with FDA approval for the treatment of tics are haloperidol, pimozide, and aripiprazole. CBIT is a first-line recommended treatment for tics; however, if tics are severely debilitating, psychopharmacology is warranted as the first-line treatment. **(pp. 445–450)**

References

American Psychiatric Association: Diagnostic and Statistical Manual of Mental Disorders, 5th Edition. Arlington, VA, American Psychiatric Association, 2013

Coffey BJ: Complexities for assessment and treatment of co-occurring ADHD and tics. Curr Dev Disord Rep 2:293–299, 2015

Darrow SM, Grados M, Sandor P, et al: Autism spectrum symptoms in a Tourette's disorder sample. J Am Acad Child Adolesc Psychiatry 56(7):610.e1–617.e1, 2017 28647013

Fernández de la Cruz L, Rydell M, Runeson B, et al: Suicide in Tourette's and chronic tic disorders. Biol Psychiatry 82(2):111–118, 2017 27773353

Hirschtritt ME, Lee PC, Pauls DL, et al: Lifetime prevalence, age of risk, and genetic relationships of comorbid psychiatric disorders in Tourette syndrome. JAMA Psychiatry 72(4):325–333, 2015 25671412

CHAPTER 21

Elimination Disorders

Wendy R. Martinez Araujo, M.D.

1.   A 6-year-old boy has been receiving outpatient treatment for enuresis for the past 6 months. His parents ask if the problem will continue when he becomes a teenager. Which of the following statements is correct?

A. There is a high rate of spontaneous remission of enuresis between ages 5 and 7 years and after age 12 years.
B. Persistence of enuresis into late adolescence is common.
C. There is a high rate of worsened symptoms around the time of puberty.
D. If enuresis is treated, it will not persist.

The correct response is Option A: There is a high rate of spontaneous remission of enuresis between ages 5 and 7 years and after age 12 years.

Typically, there is a relatively high rate of spontaneous remission between ages 5 and 7 years and after age 12 years. Yearly remission rates as high as 14%–16% have been reported (Fritz et al. 2004). Thus, enuresis is usually a self-limited disorder, and the vast majority of affected children will eventually experience spontaneous remission. The persistence of enuresis into late adolescence is rare. The treatment for enuresis, when needed, is not always successful. **(p. 461)**

2.   A 7-year-old girl is brought to the pediatric clinic after she started wetting the bed over the past 4 months, indicating secondary enuresis. Which of the following is *not* a risk factor for secondary enuresis?

A. A comorbid ADHD diagnosis.
B. Family history of enuresis.
C. Psychological stressors.
D. Nonspecific behavioral disorder.

The correct response is Option B: Family history of enuresis.

There are two subtypes of enuresis, based on the natural history of the disorder. The term *primary enuresis* is used to describe those individuals who have never achieved continence, whereas *secondary enuresis* refers to those who were able to achieve continence but then subsequently resumed wetting. A family history of enuresis is the most significant risk factor for primary enuresis. A Scandinavian epidemiological study found that the risk of enuresis for a child was 7.1 times greater if the father had enuretic events beyond age 4 (Järvelin et al. 1988).

Children with secondary enuresis are more apt to present with comorbid psychiatric disorders than are children with primary enuresis. There is a known association between enuresis and ADHD.

Additionally, children who have secondary enuresis are also more likely to have psychological stressors contributing to the loss of continence.

Other than the association of enuresis with ADHD, the primary finding in studies has been that behavioral disorders in children with enuresis are nonspecific (Mikkelsen et al. 1980). **(pp. 459, 461, 464)**

3. A 6-year-old girl who has been diagnosed with enuresis has tried various treatments without success. Of the listed medications, which would be the best option?

   A. Fluoxetine.
   B. Desvenlafaxine.
   C. Imipramine.
   D. Fluphenazine.

The correct response is Option C: Imipramine.

Imipramine is still sometimes used for children whose enuresis is refractory to other treatment methods, as either an adjunctive or a sole treatment. Multiple double-blind studies have supported imipramine use in enuresis. However, although the treatment has generally been found to be safe, there have been some tragic reports of fatal overdoses in children. Treatment guidelines for imipramine suggest cardiac monitoring and periodic testing of drug level in the blood to guard against toxicity at higher doses, as well as securing the medication against intentional or accidental overdose ingestion. For most patients, desmopressin acetate (DDAVP) is preferred as the first pharmacological option. Fluoxetine, desvenlafaxine, and fluphenazine do not have any use in enuresis. **(p. 462)**

4. What was the most significant side effect of the intranasal preparation of DDAVP, which led the FDA to issue a warning that the intranasal preparation should no longer be used for the treatment of primary nocturnal enuresis?

   A. Epistaxis.
   B. Headaches.
   C. Hyponatremia.
   D. Abdominal pain.

The correct response is Option C: Hyponatremia.

The most significant side effect that has been identified with intranasal use of DDAVP is hyponatremia and related seizures. Excess fluid intake has been identified as a contributing factor, leading to a recommendation that children do not ingest more than 8 ounces of fluid on nights when DDAVP is used (Robson et al. 1996). In recognition of the risk of hyponatremic seizures, some of which were fatal, the FDA has issued a warning that the intranasal preparation of DDAVP should no longer be used for the treatment of primary nocturnal enuresis. The most common side effects of the nasal spray formulation were abdominal pain, headaches, epistaxis, and nasal stuffiness; however, none of these led to an FDA warning. **(p. 463)**

5. A 7-year-old boy comes to the clinic accompanied by his mother. He started wetting the bed at night over the past 4 months. The mother is willing to start a behavioral treatment to stop bedwetting. What behavioral treatment has shown the same effectiveness as pharmacological treatment in enuresis?

    A. Evening fluid restriction.
    B. Retention-control training.
    C. Reward system.
    D. Bell and pad method of conditioning.

    The correct response is Option D: Bell and pad method of conditioning.

    In a large longitudinal study comparing observation only with treatment with imipramine, DDAVP, or the bell and pad method, the results clearly indicated the superiority of the bell and pad method of treatment with regard to the degree of relapse after the cessation of active treatment (Monda and Husmann 1995). Subsequent systematic reviews of the literature involving the bell and pad alarm, imipramine, and DDAVP confirmed these findings (Glazener and Evans 2002; Peng et al. 2018). The other methods have limited evidence. **(pp. 464–465)**

6. A 6-year-old boy comes to the clinic, accompanied by his parent, with a history of 5 months of defecating in his clothes. The parent reports that the boy tends to have episodes of constipation for 2–3 days in a week and afterward will defecate in his clothes. What is the best behavior-based treatment for his presentation?

    A. Bell and pad method conditioning.
    B. Daily timed intervals on the toilet with rewards.
    C. Evening restriction of food.
    D. Encouragement to use the toilets at school.

    The correct response is Option B: Daily timed intervals on the toilet with rewards.

Levine and Bakow (1976) described a treatment approach that involves educational, psychological, behavioral, and physiological components. The educational and psychological components are designed to inform the family about the functioning of the bowel and to address any interpersonal issues related to the encopresis. The physiological component involves bowel catharsis accomplished with stool softeners, enemas, and laxatives, followed by daily administration of laxatives. Daily timed intervals on the toilet, coupled with rewards for success, represent the behavioral aspects of the treatment plan. This approach continues to be a primary treatment modality. The bell and pad method of conditioning is the behavioral treatment for enuresis. Evening restriction of food or encouragement to use the toilet at school are not evidence-based behavioral treatment modalities for encopresis. **(pp. 468–469)**

References

Fritz G, Rockney R, Bernet W, et al: Practice parameter for the assessment and treatment of children and adolescents with enuresis. J Am Acad Child Adolesc Psychiatry 43(12):1540–1550, 2004 15564822

Glazener CM, Evans JH: Desmopressin for nocturnal enuresis in children. Cochrane Database Syst Rev 3(3):CD002112, 2002 12137645

Järvelin MR, Vikeväinen-Tervonen L, Moilanen I, et al: Enuresis in seven-year-old children. Acta Paediatr Scand 77(1):148–153, 1988 3369293

Levine MD, Bakow H: Children with encopresis: a study of treatment outcome. Pediatrics 58(6):845–852, 1976 995511

Mikkelsen EJ, Rapoport JL, Nee L, et al: Childhood enuresis, I: sleep patterns and psychopathology. Arch Gen Psychiatry 37(10):1139–1144, 1980 7425798

Monda JM, Husmann DA: Primary nocturnal enuresis: a comparison among observation, imipramine, desmopressin acetate and bed-wetting alarm systems. J Urol 154(2 Pt 2):745–748, 1995 7609169

Peng CC-H, Yang SS-D, Austin PF, Chang S-J: Systematic review and meta-analysis of alarm versus desmopressin therapy for pediatric monosymptomatic enuresis. Sci Rep 8(1):16755, 2018 30425276

Robson WL, Nørgaard JP, Leung AK: Hyponatremia in patients with nocturnal enuresis treated with DDAVP. Eur J Pediatr 155(11):959–962, 1996 8911897

CHAPTER 22

Sleep-Wake Disorders

Linda Schmidt, M.D.

1. With which of the following symptoms do children with narcolepsy usually present?

    A. Daytime sleepiness and sleep attacks.
    B. Excessive daytime sleepiness, cataplexy, hypnagogic hallucinations, and sleep paralysis.
    C. Excessive daytime sleepiness, hypnagogic hallucinations, and sleep paralysis.
    D. Excessive daytime sleepiness and sleep paralysis alternating with sleepwalking.

    The correct response is Option A: Daytime sleepiness and sleep attacks.

    Narcolepsy is a rare neurological disorder characterized by daytime sleepiness, cataplexy (sudden loss of muscle tone triggered by emotional arousal such as laughter), hypnagogic hallucinations, and sleep paralysis. The classic tetrad of narcolepsy that includes these symptoms is rare in children. Most pediatric patients present with excessive daytime sleepiness and sleep attacks, often masked by behavioral and emotional symptoms such as irritability, hyperactivity, inattention, and increased sleep needs. **(p. 481)**

2. Which of the following psychiatric disorders has been found to have a strong association with restless legs syndrome (RLS) or periodic limb movement disorder (PLMD)?

    A. Generalized anxiety disorder.
    B. PTSD.
    C. ADHD.
    D. Autism spectrum disorder.

    The correct response is Option C: ADHD.

A strong association between RLS, PLMD, and ADHD was found in several studies. Many children with ADHD have been found to have RLS or PLMD and vice versa.

Anxiety and sleep problems are closely tied together, especially during childhood. Although many children experience some fears at bedtime, children with anxiety disorders experience far more fear and anxiety at bedtime.

Nightmares are common in 4- to 12-year-old children; however, children exposed to major stressors, including trauma and abuse, have more persistent nightmares, frequently involving flashbacks of their traumatic experiences, with increased levels of autonomic arousal causing awakenings.

Sleep difficulties are estimated to occur in 50%–80% of children with autism spectrum disorder (Kotagal and Broomall 2012), and the most frequently reported sleep problems are bedtime resistance; difficulty falling asleep; frequent nocturnal and early morning awakenings; irregular sleep-wake cycle; restless sleep; and parasomnias such as sleepwalking, night terrors, confusional arousals, and rapid eye movement sleep behavior disorder (Diaz-Roman et al. 2018). **(pp. 485, 491–494)**

3.   When is pharmacological treatment of RLS with iron supplementation usually recommended?

A. When a child's serum ferritin level is below 25 ng/mL.
B. When a child is diagnosed with RLS.
C. When a child's serum ferritin level is below 50 ng/mL.
D. When a child's serum ferritin level is between 80 and 100 ng/mL.

The correct response is Option C: When a child's serum ferritin level is below 50 ng/mL.

Pharmacological treatment of RLS includes iron supplementation (3–6 mg/kg/day), which is usually recommended if the child's serum ferritin level is below 50 ng/mL. Serum ferritin levels should be measured every 3–4 months, with a target serum ferritin level of 80–100 ng/mL. **(p. 485)**

4.   Which of the following is required to establish a diagnosis of obstructive sleep apnea (OSA) and to assess severity and treatment efficacy?

A. Detailed sleep history and sleep diary.
B. Nocturnal polysomnography (PSG).
C. Diagnosis of adenotonsillar hypertrophy.
D. Diagnosis of adenotonsillar hypertrophy and subsequent adenotonsillectomy.

The correct response is Option B: Nocturnal polysomnography (PSG).

Nocturnal PSG is the gold standard procedure for studying sleep-disordered breathing and other types of intrinsic sleep disorders in children. The procedure involves recordings of electroencephalogram, electro-oculogram, electromyogram, airflow, respiratory and abdominal efforts, oxygen saturation, end-tidal carbon dioxide, and limb muscle activity. It requires the child and one parent or caregiver to spend a night in a sleep laboratory. PSG is indicated for diagnosing OSA, central sleep apnea, alveolar hypoventilation, snoring, and upper airway resistance syndrome in children.

Taking a sleep history is the first and most important step in assessing children and adolescents for sleep disorders. However, sleep logs are based on observations or self-perceptions and thus do not represent objective sleep assessments.

Although OSA is often the result of adenotonsillar hypertrophy, a diagnosis of adenotonsillar hypertrophy and subsequent surgical removal are not necessary to establish an OSA diagnosis. **(pp. 474–477, 486–487)**

5. Which of the following is recommended for children with OSA who either have not benefited from surgical intervention or are not candidates for surgery?

    A. Medication treatment (e.g., inhaled nasal steroids, antihistamines, nonsteroidal anti-inflammatory drugs)
    B. Continuous positive airway pressure (CPAP).
    C. Supplemental oxygen.
    D. Adenotonsillectomy.

The correct response is Option B: Continuous positive airway pressure (CPAP).

The treatment of choice for pediatric OSA is surgery, typically adenotonsillectomy; however, CPAP is recommended for children who either did not benefit from surgical intervention or are not candidates for surgery. CPAP has been approved by the FDA for use in children ages 7 years and older who weigh more than 40 pounds.

Children with allergic rhinitis and/or sinusitis may benefit from treatment with inhaled nasal steroids, antihistamines, and/or leukotriene modifiers, such as montelukast.

Supplemental oxygen is not recommended for routine use in children with OSA because of the risks of developing hypoventilation. **(p. 487)**

6. Which of the following statements regarding parasomnias is true?

    A. They occur only during slow-wave sleep.
    B. They are much more frequently seen in adults than in children.
    C. They usually worsen during adolescence.
    D. They never cause sleep disruption.

The correct response is Option A: They occur only during slow-wave sleep.

Parasomnias such as sleepwalking, sleep talking, night terrors, confusional arousals, and nocturnal enuresis occur during slow-wave sleep.

Parasomnias are much more frequently seen in children than in adults and usually represent the normal neurophysiology of sleep development.

These disorders usually appear around the second year of life and continue into the preschool or school-age years. Most parasomnias resolve by adolescence.

Parasomnias can be associated with severe sleep disruption and may cause significant family distress and daytime sleepiness. **(pp. 487–488)**

7.   Which of the following is the most common sleep-related symptom or condition in adolescents who use illicit drugs, alcohol, or cigarettes?

A. Delayed sleep phase syndrome.
B. Advanced sleep phase syndrome.
C. Sleepwalking.
D. Nightmares.

The correct response is Option A: Delayed sleep phase syndrome.

Sleep problems are highly prevalent among adolescents who use illicit drugs, alcohol, or cigarettes. The most common sleep-related symptoms among adolescents who abuse substances are excessive daytime sleepiness, insomnia, and delayed sleep phase syndrome. Advanced sleep phase syndrome is most common in preschoolers. Sleepwalking is most prevalent in children ages 4–12 years, and the peak age of nightmares is 3–6 years. **(pp. 488–490, 493)**

References

Diaz-Roman A, Zhang J, Delorme R, et al: Sleep in youth with autism spectrum disorders: systematic review and meta-analysis of subjective and objective studies. Evid Based Ment Health 21(4):146–154, 2018 30361331
Kotagal S, Broomall E: Sleep in children with autism spectrum disorder. Pediatr Neurol 47(4):242–251, 2012 22964437

CHAPTER 23

Evidence-Based Practice

John Hamilton, M.D., M.Sc.

Eric Daleiden, Ph.D.

Eric Youngstrom, Ph.D.

1. The base rate of a disorder used in Bayesian diagnostic approaches refers to which of the following?

    A. The prevalence of the disorder in the population.
    B. The prevalence of the disorder in the population adjusted for age and gender.
    C. The prevalence of the disorder in the clinic population.
    D. The lowest estimate of the disorder in the clinic population.

    The correct response is Option C: The prevalence of the disorder in the clinic population.

    Evidence-based assessment often starts with broad measures of major problem dimensions. The next assessment findings raise or lower the probability of a diagnosis until it is either functionally ruled out or clearly established as a treatment target. The most formal way of combining the information is via Bayes's theorem to integrate base rates and clinical impressions with the diagnostic likelihood ratios attached to the assessment results or clinical findings. In other words, knowing the base rates of common disorders—the proportion of all youth presenting in that clinical setting who have a specific disorder—will help clinicians calibrate diagnoses and case formulations. **(pp. 505–506)**

2.   According to Fixsen et al. (2005), which experience is essential for transferring skills from training experiences to patient interventions?

A. Studying recordings of oneself doing interventions with patients.
B. Supervision with experts trained in evidence-based treatment.
C. Peer supervision in a team setting led by an expert.
D. On-the-job coaching.

The correct response is Option D: On-the-job coaching.

Selecting a good treatment is not the same as doing a treatment well. The litmus test for treatment implementation is whether an independent observer of a session can detect the evidence-based activities as per Fixsen et al. (2005), who reviewed striking evidence that on-the-job coaching is essential to generalizing behavior from training to actual intervention sessions. **(p. 511)**

3.   Which of the following is not true regarding evidence-based practice (EBP)?

A. Even though EBP is a helpful tool, decisions about health care are based on the clinician's experience, regardless of the evidence base.
B. Decisions regarding treatment should be made by those receiving care, informed by the tacit and explicit knowledge of those providing care, within the context of available resources.
C. Loyalty to the status quo or use of merely available options, performed without measuring outcomes and implementation, is the opposite of EBP.
D. The singular term *evidence-based practice* refers to practice based on established processes for clinical decision making. The plural term *evidence-based practices* refers to those processes that are woven together to create EBP.

The correct response is Option A: Even though EBP is a helpful tool, decisions about health care are based on the clinician's experience, regardless of the evidence base.

EBP is a process in which "decisions about health care are based on the best available, current, valid and relevant evidence. These decisions should be made by those receiving care, informed by the tacit and explicit knowledge of those providing care, within the context of available resources" (Dawes et al. 2005, p. 4). The singular term refers to practice based on evidence-based processes for making clinical decisions. The plural term refers to those processes that are woven together to create EBP. EBP can also be defined by what it is not: loyalty to the status quo or use of merely available options, performed without measuring outcomes and implementation. **(p. 503)**

4. Which of the following is not in line with the principle of engaging patients and families with EBP?

A. Integrating evidence-based content into the initial contact between potential patients and care systems can create demand for EBPs and promote a match between patient characteristics and effective treatments.
B. Youth and families may help maintain EBPs by asking for and expecting services supported by evidence when they arrive at clinicians' offices.
C. The best way to engage patients and families is to not introduce EBP principles early because that may confuse them.
D. During orientation to clinical care, patients and families are encouraged to bring their own experiences and knowledge base to the evaluation process. This indicates respect for families as the experts on their own experiences, values, preferences, and history.

The correct response is Option C: The best way to engage patients and families is to not introduce EBP principles early because that may confuse them.

Integrating evidence-based content into the initial contact between potential patients and care systems can create demand for EBPs and promote a match between patient characteristics and effective treatments. For example, some clinics offer an orientation session for parents before their child sees a clinician. The orientation explains policies, educates and motivates parents and adolescents, shapes expectations, and explains treatment modalities available for common disorders. Youth and families may then help maintain EBPs by asking for and expecting services supported by evidence when they arrive at clinicians' offices. Such an orientation can also emphasize the value of patients bringing their own experiences and knowledge base to the evaluation process. It also indicates respect for families as the experts on their own experiences, values, preferences, and history. There is no evidence that introducing patients and families to EBP principles confuses them. **(p. 504)**

5. Which of the following is true regarding errors of commission and omission in the process of assessment?

A. Errors of commission assign invalid diagnoses. Errors of omission miss a diagnosis that should have been assigned.
B. Errors of commission miss a diagnosis, leading to no treatment of the true underlying condition. Errors of omission lead to a wrong diagnosis, leading to incorrect treatment.
C. When errors of commission occur, treatment may be provided without an appropriate informed consent process. Errors of omission refer to harm induced despite an informed consent process.
D. Errors of commission mean providing treatments that are not evidence-based and supported by research. Errors of omission mean not providing certain treatments despite the evidence.

The correct response is Option A: Errors of commission assign invalid diagnoses. Errors of omission miss a diagnosis that should have been assigned.

Errors of commission assign invalid diagnoses and lead to treatment choices with less chance of benefit while still carrying the full risk of harm. Errors of omission miss a diagnosis that leads to failure to intervene early and effectively and increase the chances of misattributing the sources of the problem to some other diagnosis or mechanism. **(p. 506)**

References

Dawes M, Summerskill W, Glasziou P, et al: Sicily statement on evidence-based practice. BMC Med Educ 5(1):1, 2005 15634359

Fixsen D, Naoom S, Blase K, et al: Implementation Research: A Synthesis of the Literature.Tampa, University of South Florida, 2005. Available at: https://nirn.fpg.unc.edu/sites/nirn.fpg.unc.edu/files/resources/NIRN-MonographFull-01-2005.pdf. Accessed August 11, 2020.

CHAPTER 24

Child Abuse and Neglect

Paramjit T. Joshi, M.D.

Lisa M. Cullins, M.D.

Anju Hurria, M.D., M.P.H.

1. A forensic evaluation of a child who has been physically or sexually abused should be performed by which of the following individuals?

   A. The child's therapist, who has experience with trauma-focused therapy.
   B. The child's pediatrician, who evaluates many children who have experienced abuse.
   C. The child's treating psychiatrist, whom the child sees once a month.
   D. A clinician trained in forensic assessments.

   The correct response is Option D: A clinician trained in forensic assessments.

   The forensic evaluation should be performed by a clinician trained in forensic assessment; this individual should not be the physician or therapist involved in ongoing treatment. Confidentiality issues must be clarified before a forensic evaluation. The fact that an evaluation is being done for court proceedings needs to be made clear to the parents and child from the outset. **(p. 533)**

2. Which of the following factors might predict the degree of resilience in a child who has been abused?

   A. Interpersonal trust.
   B. Paternal conflicts.
   C. School violence.
   D. Living at home with parents.

The correct response is Option A: Interpersonal trust.

Daigneault et al. (2007) studied four factors that could predict the degree of resilience: interpersonal trust, maternal conflicts, family violence, and out-of-home placements. Interpersonal trust emerged as the most predictive of resilience. **(p. 532)**

3.   Child abuse induces harm in many ways and can also be fatal. What is the leading cause of death in child abuse fatalities?

   A. Burns.
   B. Fracture.
   C. Head injury.
   D. Infection.

The correct response is Option C: Head injury.

Head injuries are the leading cause of traumatic childhood death and of child abuse fatalities. Special attention needs to be paid when examining an infant or toddler for physical abuse. The term *whiplash shaken baby syndrome* describes a constellation of clinical findings in infants and toddlers, including retinal, subdural, or subarachnoid hemorrhages, with little or no evidence of external cranial trauma. It is postulated that whiplash forces cause subdural hematomas by tearing cortical bridging veins. Serious injuries in infants are rarely accidental unless there is a clear explanation. **(p. 520)**

4.   Characteristics of sexual abuse related to poor outcomes include which of the following?

   A. Longer duration, use of force, penetration, and a perpetrator who is close or related to the child.
   B. Longer duration, use of force, penetration, and a perpetrator who is a stranger.
   C. Shorter duration, use of force, penetration, and a perpetrator who is close or related to the child.
   D. Shorter duration, use of force, penetration, and a perpetrator who is a stranger.

The correct response is Option A: Longer duration, use of force, penetration, and a perpetrator who is close or related to the child.

The data from the National Survey of Child and Adolescent Well-Being that studied children in investigations as potential victims of sexual abuse were analyzed not only for abuse rates but also for characteristics of abuse (e.g., penetration) and co-occurring family problems (McCrae et al. 2006). According to these data, characteristics of sexual abuse related to poor outcomes included longer duration, use of force, penetration, and a perpetrator who is close to or related to the child. **(p. 523)**

5.   Child neglect is a different issue from child abuse. Which of the following describes or indicates child neglect?

A. The child has a nonaccidental injury.
B. Responsible caretaking adults fail to provide adequate physical care and supervision.
C. The child has been subjected to inappropriate physical touching.
D. Abuse has been perpetrated on a teenager rather than a child.

The correct response is Option B: Responsible caretaking adults fail to provide adequate physical care and supervision.

In the Child Abuse Prevention, Adoption, and Family Services Act of 1988, *physical abuse* was defined as "the physical injury of a child under 18 years of age by a person who is responsible for the child's welfare, under circumstances which indicate that the child's health or welfare is harmed or threatened" (Kaplan et al. 1998). For the National Incidence Study, physical abuse was defined as a child younger than age 18 years experiencing nonaccidental injury (harm standard) or risk of injury (endangerment standard) as a result of having been hit with a hand or other object or having been kicked, shaken, thrown, burned, stabbed, or choked by a parent or parent substitute (Sedlak and Broadhurst 1996). *Child neglect* is differentiated from child abuse and refers to the failure of the responsible caretaking adults to provide adequate physical care and supervision. **(p. 517)**

6.   Most experts believe that physical and sexual abuse result from a combination of factors that can be categorized into those related to families and those related to the child. Which of the following is a risk factor in the child that predisposes the child to being abused?

A. Obesity.
B. Educational status.
C. Geographical location.
D. Intellectual disability.

The correct response is Option D: Intellectual disability.

Most experts believe that physical and sexual abuse result from a combination of factors within both parents and children, often in multiproblem families with significant instability.

Important family risk factors include parental mental illness or substance abuse, lack of social support, poverty, minority ethnicity, presence of four or more children in a family, young parental age, parental history of abuse, stressful events, and exposure to family violence (Chemtob et al. 2013). Although sexual abuse is prevalent in all socioeconomic classes, physical abuse and neglect may be more common in lower socioeconomic classes. However, abusers have racial, religious, and ethnic distributions similar to those of the general population (Fergusson et al. 1996; Ryan 2000).

Risk factors in the child include prematurity, intellectual disability, and physical disabilities (Cicchetti and Toth 1995). **(p. 519)**

References

Chemtob CM, Gudiño OG, Laraque D: Maternal posttraumatic stress disorder and depression in pediatric primary care: association with child maltreatment and frequency of child exposure to traumatic events. JAMA Pediatr 167(11):1011–1018, 2013 23999612

Cicchetti D, Toth SL: A developmental psychopathology perspective on child abuse and neglect. J Am Acad Child Adolesc Psychiatry 34(5):541–565, 1995 7775351

Daigneault I, Hébert M, Tourigny M: Personal and interpersonal characteristics related to resilient developmental pathways of sexually abused adolescents. Child Adolesc Psychiatr Clin N Am 16(2):415–434, 2007 17349516

Fergusson DM, Horwood LJ, Lynskey MT: Childhood sexual abuse and psychiatric disorder in young adulthood II: psychiatric outcomes of childhood sexual abuse. J Am Acad Child Adolesc Psychiatry 35(10):1365–1374, 1996 8885591

Kaplan SJ, Pelcovitz D, Salzinger S, et al: Adolescent physical abuse: risk for adolescent psychiatric disorders. Am J Psychiatry 155(7):954–959, 1998 9659863

McCrae JS, Chapman MV, Christ SL: Profile of children investigated for sexual abuse: association with psychopathology symptoms and services. Am J Orthopsychiatry 76(4):468–481, 2006 17209715

Ryan G: Childhood sexuality: a decade of study part I—research and curriculum development. Child Abuse Negl 24(1):33–48, 2000 10660008

Sedlak AJ, Broadhurst DD: The Third National Incidence Study of Child Abuse and Neglect. Washington, DC, U.S. Department of Health and Human Services, 1996

CHAPTER 25

Cultural and Religious Issues

Mary Lynn Dell, M.D., D.Min.

1.   The term *ethnicity* refers to which of the following?

   A. The physical, biological, and genetic qualities of humans.
   B. An individual's spiritual and religious beliefs only.
   C. An individual's identity with a group of people sharing common origins, customs, and beliefs.
   D. The country of one's birth and its international political positions.

   The correct response is Option C: An individual's identity with a group of people sharing common origins, customs, and beliefs.

   Ethnicity encompasses shared origins, customs, and beliefs. *Race* refers to the physical, biological, and genetic qualities of individuals. Religion and spirituality alone do not define one's ethnicity. The country where an individual is born and that nation's politics are not the same as shared origins, customs, and beliefs; ethnicity may extend beyond and is not limited to national borders and governmental jurisdictions. **(p. 540)**

2.   Which of the following best describes the concept of *religious fundamentalism*?

   A. Fluctuating beliefs of a spiritual nature, independent of the teachings, values, and behavioral expectations of specific religions and religious organizations.
   B. Strict interpretation of sacred writings and lifestyle practices guided by religious teachings that may be found worldwide in many major faith traditions.
   C. A philosophy of life that addresses life's most common, basic questions.
   D. Embracing modernity and new, popular spiritual concepts with enthusiasm.

The correct response is Option B: Strict interpretation of sacred writings and lifestyle practices guided by religious teachings that may be found worldwide in many major faith traditions.

Fundamentalism includes strict interpretation of sacred texts and lifestyle practices guided by religious teachings and is found in many major faith traditions worldwide. Fundamentalism, regardless of the major world faith tradition in which it is based, tends to be fixed, sometimes rigid, and reflects an individual's or group's understandings of the teachings and expected behaviors of religions and religious organizations. Fundamentalism is not about fluctuating beliefs of a spiritual nature, independent of the teachings, values, and behavioral expectations of specific religions and religious organizations. *Worldview*, or *Weltanschauung*, is one's philosophy of life that addresses life's most common, basic questions. Fundamentalism typically shuns modernity and developing elements of contemporary spirituality. **(pp. 543–544)**

3. A child and adolescent psychiatrist is caring for two different families who self-report membership and regular church attendance in the same Protestant denomination. One set of parents eschews premarital sex and all drug and alcohol use and insists that their children attend all of the youth activities at their church. The other set of parents states that they assume their children will be sexually active and use marijuana by the time they are in college. They permit an occasional beer on the weekends if their majority-age children will not be driving, and they did not enforce regular church attendance after their children reached high school. Which of the following is true about these families?

   A. The two families are an example of a continuum of beliefs and practices within the same and/or closely related religious denomination.
   B. Families who have religious beliefs belong to organized religious communities, so there is no need for a mental health clinician to understand the role those beliefs and practices play in the value systems of the parents and individual adolescent children.
   C. There is a possibility of emotional and/or physical neglect or abuse in the family that is more religiously observant and has stricter behavioral expectations for their children.
   D. There is a possibility of emotional and/or physical neglect or abuse in the family that is less religiously observant and has more lenient behavioral expectations for their children

The correct response is Option A: The two families are an example of a continuum of beliefs and practices within the same and/or closely related religious denomination.

There is often a continuum of beliefs and practices within the same and/or very similar denominations or faith traditions, especially regarding social issues relevant to parenting adolescents, such as sexuality, alcohol, and other substance use. Understanding the influence of religious and spiritual beliefs and practices on parenting and adolescent behaviors is always helpful, regardless of the level of religious or spiritual observance of the family or community. Clinicians must assess the risk of emotional and physical neglect or abuse on a case-by-case basis for all families, without preformed opinions based solely on the nature and extent of religious beliefs and practices. **(pp. 544–546)**

4.   Which of the following is true regarding resources helpful for patients and families that are available through local religious institutions and faith-based organizations?

A. Child and adolescent psychiatrists should avoid collaborations with religious professionals, including hospital chaplains and clergy leaders in community churches, synagogues, mosques, and other houses of worship.
B. Religious/spiritual professionals and organizations have limited interest in medical care, health, and wellness, so there is no reason to seek resources for families from religious or faith-based organizations.
C. The need for assistance from faith-based organizations and religious communities has decreased greatly in recent years because health insurance and various secular treatment programs have multiplied and become less expensive.
D. Common resources available through religious groups and faith-based organizations include food pantries, clothes closets, shelters, health clinics, transportation to medical appointments, and daycare for young children.

The correct response is Option D: Common resources available through religious groups and faith-based organizations include food pantries, clothes closets, shelters, health clinics, transportation to medical appointments, and daycare for young children.

Local religious institutions and faith-based organizations may offer food, clothing, shelter, health services, transportation, daycare for young children and the elderly, recreational opportunities, and other services that patients and their families value and find to be helpful. Child and adolescent psychiatrists and clergy alike typically value collaborative relationships with each other. Medical and religious professionals and faith-based organizations value physical and emotional health and wellness and commonly share expertise and resources in the best interests of child psychiatric patients and families. Because community services and insurance coverage for psychiatric care have decreased in recent years, the programs and resources offered by religious institutions and faith-based organizations have become even more helpful to patients and families and more highly appreciated by the mental health clinicians who care for them. **(p. 547)**

5.   The DSM-5 section "Cultural Formulation" (American Psychiatric Association 2013) includes which of the following?

A. Only a limited description of physical and emotional symptoms commonly experienced by refugees fleeing from specific countries.
B. No consideration of the ways suffering is communicated by individuals from diverse cultural groups.
C. Suggested outlines for inclusion of relevant information about cultural identity, cultural understandings of distress, psychosocial stressors and cultural features of vulnerability and resilience, and cultural understandings of the relationships between individuals and clinicians.
D. No information helpful for understanding children and adolescents younger than 18 years of age and their families.

The correct response is Option C: Suggested outlines for inclusion of relevant information about cultural identity, cultural understandings of distress, psychosocial stressors and cultural features of vulnerability and resilience, and cultural understandings of the relationships between individuals and clinicians.

The DSM-5 "Cultural Formulation" section provides information and suggested interview items helpful to practicing clinicians, including questions related to cultural identity, understanding of distress, psychosocial stressors and cultural understandings of vulnerability and resilience, and effective therapeutic relationships. *Cultural syndromes* are consistent physical and emotional symptoms that occur in cultural groups or contexts and are insufficient for a cultural formulation. The understanding and expression of suffering by individuals from diverse cultural groups, known as the *cultural idiom of distress*, are also insufficient to stand alone as a cultural formulation. Information derived from the DSM-5 Cultural Formulation can be very useful for understanding children, adolescents, their families, significant adults in children's lives, and cultural aspects of their care. **(p. 542)**

Reference

American Psychiatric Association: Diagnostic and Statistical Manual of Mental Disorders, 5th Edition. Arlington, VA, American Psychiatric Association, 2013

CHAPTER 26

Youth Suicide

David A. Brent, M.D.

Tina R. Goldstein, Ph.D.

Craig J.R. Sewall, Ph.D., LCSW

1. Sam, a 16-year-old boy, decides late one evening that he is going to kill himself to "end the pain." He grabs a bottle of pills from the bathroom and unscrews the cap, but before he is able to put any pills in his mouth, his mother knocks on the door. Sam puts the pills away and goes to bed. How should this event be classified?

    A. Suicide attempt.
    B. Interrupted suicide attempt.
    C. Aborted suicide attempt.
    D. Nonsuicidal self-injurious behavior.

    The correct response is Option B: Interrupted suicide attempt.

    Because Sam did not actually ingest any pills, this event should not be considered a suicide attempt. Sam started to make a suicide attempt but was interrupted by another person prior to experiencing any injury, so this event should be considered an interrupted suicide attempt. Sam was interrupted by another person rather than stopping himself before experiencing any injury, so this event should not be considered an aborted suicide attempt; in an aborted suicide attempt, the person begins to make a suicide attempt but stops themselves prior to experiencing an injury. Sam retrieved the pills with the intention of killing himself, and he did not experience any injury, so this event should not be considered nonsuicidal self-injurious behavior. **(p. 552, Table 26–1).**

2.   Which of the following statements regarding suicidal thoughts and behaviors among male versus female youth is correct?

A. The rate of death by suicide is higher for female youth than male youth.
B. Male youth endorse higher rates of suicidal ideation than do female youth.
C. The rate of attempted suicide is higher for female youth than male youth.
D. Compared with cisgender youth, transgender youth are less likely to ideate and attempt suicide.

The correct response is Option C: The rate of attempted suicide is higher for female youth than male youth.

Even though female youth attempt suicide at a higher rate than do male youth (Ruch et al. 2019) and female youth endorse higher rates of suicidal ideation than do male youth (Centers for Disease Control and Prevention 2017), male youth are more likely to die by suicide (Hedegaard et al. 2018). The higher rate of deaths by suicide among male youth may be attributable to higher rates of associated risk factors, including substance use and antisocial behaviors, and the tendency for male youth to use more violent and lethal means when attempting suicide. Compared with cisgender youth, transgender youth are much more likely to ideate and attempt suicide (Thoma et al. 2019). Similarly, compared with heterosexual youth, sexual minority youth are at substantially greater risk of suicidal ideation (47.7% vs. 13.3%) and attempted suicide (23.0% vs. 5.4%) (Centers for Disease Control and Prevention 2017). **(p. 552)**

3.   Approximately ____ of youth with suicidal ideation go on to attempt suicide.

A. 50%.
B. 10%.
C. 25%.
D. 33%.

The correct response is Option D: 33%.

According to a nationally representative study (Nock et al. 2013), about one-third of youth with suicidal ideation go on to make a suicide plan, and about one-third of those with suicidal ideation attempt suicide. **(p. 553)**

4.   Suicidal ideation should be assessed according to both severity (intent) and pervasiveness (frequency and intensity). Which of the following is *not* one of the four components of suicidal intent that should be explored?

A. Extent to which the person wants to die.
B. Preparatory behaviors.
C. Prevention of discovery.
D. Prior history of suicidal behavior.

The correct response is Option D: Prior history of suicidal behavior.

Even though it is important to assess the person's prior history of suicidal behavior during a suicide risk assessment, this is not one of the four components of suicidal intent. The four components of suicidal intent that should be explored are 1) belief about intent (i.e., the extent to which the person wants to die), 2) preparatory behaviors (e.g., giving away prized possessions or writing a suicide note), 3) prevention of discovery (i.e., planning the attempt so that rescue is unlikely), and 4) communication of suicidal intent. High intent—as evidenced by expressing a wish to die, planning the attempt ahead of time, timing the attempt to avoid detection, and confiding suicide plans prior to the attempt—is associated with recurrent suicide attempts and death from suicide. **(p. 555)**

5.   Which of the following risk factors is the strongest predictor of future suicidal behavior?

A. Previous self-injurious behavior.
B. Having a mood disorder.
C. Family history of suicidal behavior.
D. Having a chronic medical condition.

The correct response is Option A: Previous self-injurious behavior.

According to a meta-analysis of 50 years of research on suicidal thoughts and behavior (Franklin et al. 2016), previous self-injurious behavior—including a history of prior attempts and/or a history of nonsuicidal self-injury—was the strongest predictor of future suicidal behavior. **(p. 553)**

6.   All of the following are evidence-based approaches to clinical management of youth suicidality except

A. Safety plans.
B. Means restriction.
C. Inpatient hospitalization.
D. Cognitive-behavioral therapy.

The correct response is Option C: Inpatient hospitalization.

Although psychiatric hospital admission is believed to be useful in safely resolving acute suicidal crises, there is no research on its efficacy. Safety planning is considered best practice for suicide prevention with at-risk individuals. Evidence suggests that restricting access to lethal means of suicide is an effective suicide prevention tool. In particular, the removal of guns from the homes of at-risk youth is strongly recommended. Several research studies suggest that cognitive-behavioral therapy is associated with reductions in suicidality. **(pp. 556–558)**

References

Centers for Disease Control and Prevention: Youth Risk Behavior Survey: Data Summary and Trends Report. Atlanta, GA, Centers for Disease Control and Prevention, 2017. Available at: https://www.cdc.gov/healthyyouth/data/yrbs/pdf/trendsreport.pdf. Accessed October 6, 2020.

Franklin JC, Ribeiro JD, Fox KR, et al: Risk factors for suicidal thoughts and behaviors: a meta-analysis of 50 years of research. Psychol Bull 143(2):187–232, 2016 27841450

Hedegaard H, Curtin SC, Warner M: Suicide mortality in the United States, 1999–2017. NCHS Data Brief No 330, November 2018. Available at: https://www.cdc.gov/nchs/data/databriefs/db330_tables-508.pdf#2. Accessed October 6, 2020.

Nock MK, Green JG, Hwang I, et al: Prevalence, correlates, and treatment of lifetime suicidal behavior among adolescents: results from the National Comorbidity Survey Replication Adolescent Supplement. JAMA Psychiatry 70(3):300–310, 2013 23303463

Ruch DA, Sheftall AH, Schlagbaum P, et al: Trends in suicide among youth aged 10 to 19 years in the United States, 1975 to 2016. JAMA Netw Open 2(5):e193886, 2019 31099867

Thoma BC, Salk RH, Choukas-Bradley S, et al: Suicidality disparities between transgender and cisgender adolescents. Pediatrics 144(5):e20191183, 2019 31611339

C H A P T E R 2 7

Gender and Sexual Diversity in Childhood and Adolescence

Jonathon Wanta, M.D.

Briahna Yuodsnukis, Ph.D.

Aron Janssen, M.D.

1.   A 12-year-old nonbinary individual presents to your clinic for an initial assessment. They report 6 months of increasing anxiety and social isolation. Which of the following should be considered in assessing and formulating this patient?

A. Bullying at school due to their nonbinary identity.
B. Fear of rejection by friends and family.
C. Baseline social anxiety.
D. All of the above.

The correct response is Option D: All of the above.

LGBTQ+ individuals may identify one or more factors contributing to their psychopathology. Like their cisgender heterosexual peers, they may exhibit psychopathology independent of their LGBTQ+ identity (e.g., general mood concerns). They may also experience symptoms secondary to discrimination and bias because of their LGBTQ+ identity (e.g., bullying, rejection by peers and family) and/or psychopathology resulting from internalized rejection and shame about their LGBTQ+ identity (e.g., negative expectations about the future, fear of future rejection or victimization). Clinicians should assess all factors contributing to the patient's presentation to assist in case formulation and treatment. **(pp. 569–570)**

2. Which of the following describes how cumulative exposure to external stressors (such as bullying) and internal stressors (such as internalized homophobia) increases the risk of adverse mental and physical health outcomes?

A. Minority stress theory.
B. Transactional theory of stress and coping.
C. Overcoming adversity theory.
D. General adaptation syndrome.

The correct response is Option A: Minority stress theory.

Minority stress theory was adapted for sexual minorities by Meyer (2003) and for gender minorities by Hendricks and Testa (2012). This theory describes how experiences of external stressors (e.g., discrimination, victimization, rejection, nonaffirmation) and internal stressors (e.g., internalized stigma, negative expectations of the future, concealment) increase the risk of adverse mental and physical health outcomes for gender and sexual minorities.

The transactional theory of stress and coping was proposed by Lazarus and Folkman (1984). This model has been adapted to understand stressors related to discrimination and stigma, but it emphasizes appraisals of threat and harm more broadly.

The general adaptation syndrome (Selye 1950) describes the body's response to stress. **(p. 570)**

3. Which of the following medical and surgical treatments is considered *fully reversible* for transgender and nonbinary youth?

A. Puberty blockers.
B. Gender-affirming testosterone therapy.
C. Gender-affirming estrogen therapy.
D. Vaginoplasty.

The correct response is Option A: Puberty blockers.

Puberty blockers are generally seen as a reversible medical intervention. Puberty blockers suspend pubertal development by preventing the production of gonadal sex hormones. This medication can provide youth with time to mature and consider whether they would like to pursue other gender-affirming medical interventions that may be irreversible. Gender-diverse youth can discontinue puberty blockers without experiencing permanent changes. Gender-affirming hormone therapies are *partially irreversible* because there may be both reversible and irreversible changes. For example, testosterone therapy may lead to a permanent deepening of the voice, but fat distribution and muscle mass may return to the preintervention baseline once testosterone is discontinued. Surgical interventions are generally considered fully irreversible. **(p. 575)**

4. Most children can have a basic understanding of gender by what age?

A. 1 year.
B. 3 years.
C. 7 years.
D. 12 years.

The correct response is Option B: 3 years.

By age 2–3 years, children often have a basic understanding of gender and gender roles, including use of gendered pronouns and recognition of gender differences. Most children this age are able to label their own gender, although this is often limited to "boy" or "girl." By age 5–7 years, most children have developed an internal sense of gender that is consistent across time and situations. Nevertheless, there may be variability and exploration at this age. A person's understanding of gender will continue to evolve throughout adolescence and young adulthood. **(p. 567)**

5. Which of the following psychotherapeutic interventions is *not* recommended for transgender and gender nonbinary youth?

A. Adapting evidence-based interventions to target minority stress sequelae.
B. Cognitive-behavioral therapy (CBT) to change the patient's gender identity.
C. Collaborating with and providing psychoeducation to families.
D. Advocating for equitable and nondiscriminatory policies at school.

The correct response is Option B: Cognitive-behavioral therapy (CBT) to change the patient's gender identity.

A clinician should never try to change a person's gender identity; doing so can cause significant harm and is unethical. LGBTQ+ youth often face unique stressors that can influence mental health and well-being. Although no randomized controlled trials of interventions are currently designed specifically for LGBTQ+ youth, adapting current evidence-based treatment may be effective. Clinicians can support LGBTQ+ youth in many other ways that can promote resiliency factors, such as community connectedness and support. CBT may be used to provide an LGBTQ+ young person with skills to cope with distress rather than challenging their gender identity. **(pp. 571, 573–574)**

6. Which of the following questions is the most appropriate for assessing sexual orientation?

A. Have you ever had a boyfriend?
B. Are you romantically attracted to any peers at school?
C. Are you romantically attracted to boys or girls?
D. There is no need to ask because sexual minority patients will bring it up without prompting if it is important.

The correct response is Option B: Are you romantically attracted to any peers at school?

Questions regarding gender and sexuality historically have been discussed in binary contexts (e.g., "Are you a boy or a girl?" or "Are you attracted to boys or girls?"). Many youth may have identities that do not fit within the binary system. Open-ended questions should be used to allow youth to provide responses based on their personal experiences. Closed-ended or binary questions may invalidate or discredit a young person's experience if they do not fit within those categories. It is important to assess sexuality at developmentally appropriate levels because it may provide information about the youth's social system. For LGBTQ+ youth, asking questions may elicit conversations about sexuality that may not be discussed otherwise or provide the clinical opportunity to identify possible support needed. **(p. 572)**

7.   Which of the following publishes standards of care for clinicians in evaluating and managing transgender and gender-diverse individuals?

A. The World Professional Association of Transgender Health (WPATH).
B. The Trevor Project.
C. The Family Acceptance Project.
D. Parents, Families, and Friends of Lesbians and Gays (PFLAG).

The correct response is Option A: The World Professional Association of Transgender Health (WPATH).

WPATH is an organization that publishes recommendations for evidence-based assessments and interventions for transgender and gender-diverse individuals (Coleman et al. 2012). The other options refer to LGBTQ+-affirmative organizations that may be useful sources of support and resources for LGBTQ+ youth and their families and support systems. **(p. 573)**

References

Coleman E, Bockting W, Botzer M, et al: Standards of Care for the Health of Transsexual, Transgender, and Gender-Nonconforming People, Version 7. Int J Transgend 13(4):165–232, 2012
Hendricks ML, Testa RJ: A conceptual framework for clinical work with transgender and gender nonconforming clients: an adaptation of the minority stress model. Prof Psychol Res Pract 43(5):460–467, 2012
Lazarus RS, Folkman S: Stress, Appraisal and Coping. New York, Springer, 1984
Meyer IH: Prejudice, social stress, and mental health in lesbian, gay, and bisexual populations: conceptual issues and research evidence. Psychol Bull 129(5):674–697, 2003 12956539
Selye H: Stress and the general adaptation syndrome. Br Med J 1(4667):1383–1392, 1950 15426759

CHAPTER 28

Aggression and Violence

Jeffrey H. Newcorn, M.D.

Yael Kufert, M.D.

Iliyan Ivanov, M.D.

Anil Chacko, Ph.D.

1. What is the relationship between alcohol and drug use disorders and aggression?

    A. Alcohol and drug use disorders are not associated with increased odds of aggression.
    B. Alcohol use disorder is not associated with increased odds of aggression, but drug use disorders are.
    C. Drug use disorders are not associated with increased odds of aggression, but alcohol use disorder is.
    D. Both alcohol use disorder and drug use disorders are associated with significantly increased odds of aggression toward self and others.

    The correct response is Option D: Both alcohol use disorder and drug use disorders are associated with significantly increased odds of aggression toward self and others.

    The use of alcohol and drugs is associated with an increased risk of aggression directed at both self and others. The association is through the direct effect of substances as well as through shared risk factors predisposing the user to substance abuse and aggression. **(p. 583)**

2.   Which of the following statements regarding aggression and violence is the most accurate?

A. Aggression and violence among youth are rare and do not represent a major public health concern.
B. A temporary decrease in similar events often occurs over the 2 weeks following a mass school shooting.
C. School shootings are less likely to occur in states with higher mental health expenditures.
D. A temporary increase in similar events often occurs over the 2 months following a mass school shooting.

The correct response is Option C: School shootings are less likely to occur in states with higher mental health expenditures.

State-level risk factors associated with school shootings include lower mental health expenditures and a higher prevalence of firearm ownership (Kalesan et al. 2017). An element of contagion is often seen in school shootings; specifically, a temporary increase in similar events occurs immediately following a mass shooting over the 2 weeks, not 2 months, following such an event (Towers et al. 2015). **(p. 582)**

3.   In neuroimaging studies, abnormal gray matter volumes in which of the following brain regions is found to be associated with aggressive behaviors?

A. Ventral striatum.
B. Insula.
C. Dorsolateral prefrontal cortex.
D. Cerebellum.

The correct response is Option B: Insula.

Findings from neuroimaging studies have shown that, in comparison with healthy control subjects, adolescents with conduct disorder and aggressive behaviors exhibit abnormal gray matter volumes in the frontal and parietal lobes (which inhibit limbic and other subcortical regions), anterior cingulate cortex (which manages incoming affective stimuli), and insula (which integrates emotion and cognitive processing) (Zhang et al. 2018). The ventral striatum has been implicated in reward processing, specifically with reward anticipation. The dorsolateral prefrontal cortex is implicated in top-down regulatory control of behavior. The cerebellum is hypothesized to play a role in motor learning. **(pp. 583–584)**

4.   Which neurochemical has been associated with the development of antisocial personality disorder (ASPD) in late adolescence to early adulthood for boys?

A. Dopamine.
B. Testosterone.

C. Serotonin.

D. Glutamate.

The correct response is Option C: Serotonin.

A study revealed that low CNS serotonin (as indexed by prolactin or cortisol release after fenfluramine challenge) at ages 7–11 years was associated with increased aggression in adolescence and also was associated with heightened risk for ASPD and borderline personality disorder in middle to late adolescence (on average, 9 years later) and early adulthood (on average, 15 years later) (Flory et al. 2007). No reports show that the other neurochemicals have predictive value in ASPD development, although many neurochemicals are implicated in aggression and violence in general. **(p. 584)**

5. Which of the following is true when more intensive antibullying programs are compared with less intensive ones?

    A. Both have similar outcomes.
    B. Better outcomes are found with more intensive programs.
    C. Poorer outcomes are found with more intensive programs.
    D. Insufficient data are available to compare varying intensities of antibullying programs.

The correct response is Option B: Better outcomes are found with more intensive programs.

School antibullying programs have received attention over the past few years and share many features with other school-based violence prevention programs (e.g., a focus on knowledge, attitude change, monitoring of behavior in school, and discipline methods). Overall, data suggest that antibullying programs can decrease bullying in schools by 23% and victimization by 20% (Farrington et al. 2017; Jiménez-Barbero et al. 2016; Lee et al. 2015). More intensive antibullying programs that include certain key features (e.g., parent meetings, firm disciplinary methods, improved playground supervision) result in better outcomes (Ttofi and Farrington 2011). Although antibullying programs vary in intensity (duration, specificity, and components), there is a generally positive relationship between intensity and outcomes. **(pp. 589–590)**

6. A meta-analysis of studies of parent training programs (Wyatt Kaminski et al. 2008) found that all of the following are commonly used and effective aspects of parenting interventions for preventing aggressive behavior except

    A. Increasing positive parent-child interactions.
    B. Increasing parenting consistency.
    C. Behavioral reward systems.
    D. Problem-solving skills.

The correct response is Option D: Problem-solving skills.

Although problem-solving skills for both parents and children are part of some parenting interventions, the findings relevant to added value of this component are equivocal. However, all parenting interventions that effectively address aggressive behavior in children include the following: positive parent-child interactions, parent consistency with consequences, and behavioral reward systems to support behavior change. **(p. 590)**

7.   Which of the following statements regarding pharmacotherapy for aggressive behavior in children is correct?

A. Treating underlying ADHD can be a useful strategy.
B. No clinical trial data support the use of mood-stabilizing medications such as lithium and divalproex.
C. Controlled clinical trials indicate that α_2-agonists effectively treat physical aggression in the context of ADHD.
D. Risperidone is an FDA-approved treatment for aggression and should be the first medication used for this condition.

The correct response is Option A: Treating underlying ADHD can be a useful strategy.

Numerous studies show that treating underlying ADHD results in a decrease in rates of aggression.

Supportive clinical trial data are available for mood stabilizers such as lithium and divalproex.

No data show that the α_2-agonists have a positive effect on aggression, although it is presumed that they may be effective because of their effects on impulsivity. Certainly, no data indicate that the α_2-agonists are an effective treatment for physical aggression in the context of ADHD.

Risperidone has the best data for specific treatment of aggression, but it is not FDA approved for that indication. In fact, it is approved not for aggression at all but rather for irritability in autism spectrum disorder. **(pp. 596–597)**

References

Farrington DP, Gaffney H, Lösel F, Ttofi MM: Systematic reviews of the effectiveness of developmental prevention programs in reducing delinquency, aggression, and bullying. Aggress Violent Behav 33:91–106, 2017

Flory JD, Newcorn JH, Miller C, et al: Serotonergic function in children with attention-deficit hyperactivity disorder: relationship to later antisocial personality disorder. Br J Psychiatry 190:410–414, 2007 17470955

Jiménez-Barbero JA, Ruiz-Hernández JA, Llor-Zaragoza L, et al: Effectiveness of anti-bullying school programs: a meta-analysis. Child Youth Serv Rev 61:165–175, 2016

Kalesan B, Lagast K, Villarreal M, et al: School shootings during 2013–2015 in the USA. Inj Prev 23(5):321–327, 2017 27923800

Lee S, Kim C-J, Kim DH: A meta-analysis of the effect of school-based anti-bullying programs. J Child Health Care 19(2):136–153, 2015 24092871

Towers S, Gomez-Lievano A, Khan M, et al: Contagion in mass killings and school shootings. PLoS One 10(7):e0117259, 2015 26135941

Ttofi MM, Farrington DP: Effectiveness of school-based programs to reduce bullying: a systematic and meta-analytic review. J Exp Criminol 7(1):27–56, 2011

Wyatt Kaminski J, Valle LA, Filene JH, et al: A meta-analytic review of components associated with parent training program effectiveness. J Abnorm Child Psychol 36(4):567–589, 2008 18205039

Zhang J, Liu W, Zhang J, et al: Distinguishing adolescents with conduct disorder from typically developing youngsters based on pattern classification of brain structural MRI. Front Hum Neurosci 12:152, 2018 29740296

CHAPTER 29

Psychiatric Emergencies

Lisa L. Giles, M.D.

1. Which of the following tools has been validated to screen for suicide risk in a pediatric emergency department (ED) setting?

    A. Suicide Assessment Five-Step Evaluation and Triage (SAFE-T).
    B. Ask Suicide-Screening Questions (ASQ).
    C. Patient Safety Screener (PSS-3).
    D. Patient Health Questionnaire–9 (PHQ-9).

    The correct response is Option B: Ask Suicide-Screening Questions (ASQ).

    Only two screening tools have been validated in a pediatric ED setting: the ASQ (Horowitz et al. 2012) and the Risk of Suicide Questionnaire (RSQ; Horowitz et al. 2001).

    The Suicide Assessment Five-Step Evaluation and Triage (SAFE-T) was derived from data and recommendations included in the American Psychiatric Association (2003) *Practice Guideline for the Assessment and Treatment of Patients With Suicidal Behaviors*.

    The PSS-3 is a three-item screener for depression, active suicidal ideation, and prior lifetime suicide attempts that was tested in adult ED patients (Boudreaux et al. 2015).

    The PHQ-9 (Kroenke et al. 2001) was validated using a set of primary care patients and subsequently with several subpopulations, including psychiatry patients with medical comorbidities, pregnant patients, and patients evaluated in an occupational health setting. **(p. 606)**

2. A 14-year-old postmenarchal adolescent with a known history of anxiety and depression is brought to the ED by her parents after expressing suicidal ideation to her outpatient therapist. The patient denies any suicide attempts. A physical

exam is normal with no obvious signs of toxicity. Which laboratory studies would be indicated during the assessment?

A. Thyroid-stimulating hormone and free T_4.
B. Complete blood count with differential, renal panel, and liver function tests.
C. Pregnancy test.
D. Erythrocyte sedimentation rate.

The correct response is Option C: Pregnancy test.

A pregnancy test for adolescent girls and a urine toxicology screen are often indicated. The former is to prevent possible teratogenic side effects of psychotropic medications, and the latter is to detect a possible etiological factor in the development of suicidal behavior. Additional laboratory studies depend on the method of suicide attempts and resulting physical complications. Generally, unless there are obvious signs of illness, consensus guidelines state that additional medical workup is rarely needed in the emergent evaluation of the suicidal patient. **(p. 606)**

3.   An ED crisis worker assesses a 16-year-old adolescent who is presenting to the ED after posting a suicide plan on his social media account. Which of the following features, if present in the patient's current presentation or history, would best support the consulting psychiatrist's recommendation for psychiatric hospitalization?

A. The patient refuses to sign a no-suicide contract.
B. The parents are requesting an admission.
C. The patient is currently intoxicated.
D. The patient describes a specific suicide plan with clear lethality and feasibility.

The correct response is Option D: The patient describes a specific suicide plan with clear lethality and feasibility.

After assessing the patient's suicide risk factors, a recommendation for psychiatric hospitalization is made if there is evidence of strong suicidal intent. An example is a child who has frequent and long-standing thoughts of suicide and/or who describes specific plans that are not only potentially lethal but also feasible. Clinicians should be particularly concerned when the idea of suicide seems acceptable to the patient. Suicidal patients with a history of unsuccessful treatment in psychiatric outpatient or day hospital settings and/or poorly controlled substance use should also be considered for inpatient admission. Young patients who are intoxicated at ED admission should be observed and reassessed when sober. A lack of appropriate social support may indicate a need for inpatient psychiatric admission to ensure patient safety and treatment adherence. Developing a "no suicide contract" or safety plan may be a helpful exercise when planning disposition, but it is not an indicator of the patient's safety. As explained here, the decision to admit the patient depends on multiple factors, and parental request alone is not adequate. **(pp. 607–608)**

4. A 12-year-old boy is brought to the ED by the police after becoming aggressive at school. Which of the following should be included as part of the initial management in the emergency department?

    A. Administer intramuscular haloperidol and lorazepam.
    B. Place the patient in mechanical restraints.
    C. Provide a calm environment with preferred distractions while collecting additional history about triggers and helpful responses.
    D. Prepare for transfer for psychiatric hospitalization.

    The correct response is Option C: Provide a calm environment with preferred distractions while collecting additional history about triggers and helpful responses.

    Ideally, all ED staff and consultants should be skilled at recognizing the early signs of agitation and be able to intervene before symptoms escalate. Simple interventions include dimming lights, offering preferred sensory tools or distraction techniques, providing visible schedules, and avoiding unnecessary interventions (e.g., frequent vital signs checks). During interactions with irritable children and adolescents, it is helpful to stay calm and use simple language, with clinicians clearly identifying themselves, their role, and planned interventions. Body language should be respectful and nonconfrontational without sudden movement or intrusions into the patient's personal space. Providing choices (e.g., snacks, television channels) while setting clear limits can help youth feel some control.

    Most experts agree that the use of seclusion and/or restraint should be reserved for when other strategies are unsuccessful and the patient poses an imminent threat of harm to themselves or others.

    There is growing evidence to guide the use of medications in the management of agitation in the ED as one part of a comprehensive strategy to address agitated behaviors (Gerson et al. 2019). The goals of pharmacotherapy include targeting the underlying cause of distress and calming the patient sufficiently for rapid assessment and treatment. Therefore, it is important to discern the causes of the patient's agitation and select medication on the basis of the patient's specific needs and history. Medications that target the underlying illness should be used when possible.

    Although a decision to transfer to a psychiatric facility might eventually be needed, it is not appropriate as a default best next step when evaluating a patient for aggression at school. **(pp. 610–611)**

5. Which of the following is true regarding the use of antipsychotic medications to treat agitation in pediatric patients in the ED?

    A. Severe agitation, especially in the setting of delirium, psychosis, or alcohol intoxication, may indicate the use of antipsychotic medications.
    B. Combining intramuscular olanzapine with intravenous benzodiazepine when agitation is extreme is the ideal choice when medication use is necessary.

C. Intravenous ziprasidone can be used to address extreme aggression.

D. When agitation is escalating, it is appropriate to continue administering increasing dosages of antipsychotics.

The correct response is Option A: Severe agitation, especially in the setting of delirium, psychosis, or alcohol intoxication, may indicate the use of antipsychotic medications.

Antipsychotic medications should be considered for severe agitation, especially in the presence of delirium, mania, psychosis, or alcohol intoxication. Historically, haloperidol and chlorpromazine have been used, and more recently, atypical antipsychotics, especially risperidone and olanzapine, have been chosen. More sedating medications with rapid onset of action, such as olanzapine, are often preferred. Studies show the effectiveness of intramuscular olanzapine and intramuscular ziprasidone. However, the use of ziprasidone raises concerns, including its activating properties, potential risk of QT prolongation, and need for concomitant food intake when taken by mouth (Khan and Michan 2006). Olanzapine and benzodiazepines should not be administered parenterally within 1 hour of each other because of the risk of respiratory suppression. Total daily and cumulative doses should be monitored closely because medication-induced akathisia and other extrapyramidal side effects can be misperceived as worsening agitation. **(p. 612)**

6. The ED can be a particularly challenging environment for patients with autism spectrum disorder. Which of the following interventions may improve cooperation?

A. Involve the primary caregiver when communicating and negotiating with the patient.

B. Quickly introduce interventions to avoid increasing the patient's anticipatory anxiety.

C. Encourage multiple staff members to check on the patient frequently.

D. Place the patient in a room near the nurses' station so that the patient will be under constant observation and cannot leave the room for any reason.

The correct response is Option A: Involve the primary caregiver when communicating and negotiating with the patient.

ED staff ideally should provide a safe and quiet environment for patients with autism spectrum disorder that is away from traffic and where the door can close and the family can have privacy. Because the parent or primary caregiver generally understands how best to communicate with the child and establish a level of cooperation that allows for assessment and treatment, communication with autistic patients should be done through the caregiver whenever possible. The caregiver can be a source of information on the patient's needs during the ED admission, can define the parameters of calm and safe surroundings for the child, and can assist in the medical management of the patient, particularly if urgent administration of medication is needed.

For patients with autism spectrum disorder, rehearsing interventions rather than introducing them quickly may help preparation for treatment.

In the ED, clinical staff routinely check on patients who are waiting for an examination. For autistic patients, frequent interruptions can be unsettling. A small and consistent group of clinicians can develop simple, familiar routines for the patient during even brief stays in the ED. Planned breaks should be included because autistic patients may struggle to stay in one location for an extended period. These "pauses" can include distractions such as games and videos or bathroom breaks. **(pp. 614–615)**

7.   A psychiatric consultation is requested for a 14-year-old female adolescent who presents in the ED with possible psychosis. In addition to the acute onset of hallucinations, she is observed to have waxing and waning levels of disorientation and agitation. Which of the following should be part of the management of this patient in the ED?

A. Ensure that the patient's pain, if present, is adequately covered with opioid medications.
B. Consider the use of lorazepam to help manage agitation.
C. Immediately administer an antipsychotic and transfer the patient to a psychiatric hospital.
D. Offer repeated reassurance and reorientation while evaluating the patient for underlying disease processes.

The correct response is Option D: Offer repeated reassurance and reorientation while evaluating the patient for underlying disease processes.

Early recognition of delirium in the ED is critical to ensure appropriate treatment and disposition. The most effective treatment for delirium is the correction of the underlying disease process, and thus the presence of delirium, as suggested by the patient's waxing and waning levels of disorientation and agitation, should prompt a thorough medical workup. In addition, the use of medications that may be deliriogenic (especially anticholinergics, opioids, and benzodiazepines) should be minimized, and the environment should be optimized to both prevent and treat delirium. Environmental interventions include providing repeated reassurance and reorientation; decreasing stimuli; and surrounding the patient with familiar, comforting objects (Patel et al. 2017; Silver et al. 2019). When resolution of the primary cause is not immediately possible, the ED clinician may need to treat the symptoms of delirium with antipsychotic medication in order to ease distress and facilitate appropriate medical workup and subsequent care. **(p. 616)**

References

American Psychiatric Association: Practice Guideline for the Assessment and Treatment of Patients With Suicidal Behaviors. Arlington, VA, American Psychiatric Association, 2003

Boudreaux ED, Jaques ML, Brady KM, et al: The patient safety screener: validation of a brief suicide risk screener for emergency department settings. Arch Suicide Res 19(2):151–160, 2015 25826715

Gerson R, Malas N, Feuer V, et al: Best practices for evaluation and treatment of agitated children and adolescents (BETA) in the emergency department: consensus statement of the American Association for Emergency Psychiatry. West J Emerg Med 20(2):409–418, 2019 30881565

Horowitz LM, Wang PS, Koocher GP, et al: Detecting suicide risk in a pediatric emergency department: development of a brief screening tool. Pediatrics 107(5):1133–1137, 2001 11331698

Horowitz LM, Bridge JA, Teach SJ, et al: Ask Suicide-Screening Questions (ASQ): a brief instrument for the pediatric emergency department. Arch Pediatr Adolesc Med 166(12):1170–1176, 2012 23027429

Khan S, Michan L: A naturalistic evaluation of intramuscular ziprasidone versus intramuscular olanzapine for the management of acute agitation and aggression in children and adolescents. J Child Adolesc Psychopharmacol 16(6):671–677, 2006 17201611

Kroenke K, Spitzer RL, Williams JB: The PHQ-9: validity of a brief depression severity measure. J Gen Intern Med 16(9):606–613, 2001 11556941

Patel AK, Bell MJ, Traube C: Delirium in pediatric critical care. Pediatr Clin N Am 64(5):1117–1132, 2017 28941539

Silver GH, Kearney JA, Bora S, et al: A clinical pathway to standardize care of children with delirium in pediatric inpatient settings. Hosp Pediatr 9(11):909–916, 2019 31662421

CHAPTER 30

Family Transitions

Challenges and Resilience

Emanuel Martinez, M.D.

1. When multistressed families are in therapy, which of the following is a concept that seeks to empower struggling families to master the challenges in their stress-laden lives?

    A. Resilience-oriented perspective.
    B. Problem-saturated family narrative.
    C. Problem-focused therapy.
    D. Strengths-oriented assessment.

    The correct response is Option A: Resilience-oriented perspective.

    In therapy, it is crucial to understand how symptoms and catastrophic fears are fueled by overwhelming stresses, trauma, and losses. A resilience-oriented perspective seeks to empower struggling families to master the challenges of their stress-laden lives.

    Problem-saturated family narrative and problem-focused therapy are not concepts that seek to empower struggling families to master the challenges in their stress-laden lives. When therapy is overly problem focused, it grimly replicates the family's problem-saturated experience.

    A strengths-oriented assessment lays the groundwork for therapist-family collaboration by prioritizing areas of concern and identifying potential resources in kin and community networks. **(pp. 631–632)**

2.	In Falicov's multilevel model for prevention and intervention with transnational families, which of the following refers to the relational context?

A. The loss of social networks.
B. Issues of cultural diversity.
C. Reconstitution of old and new community bonds.
D. Marital and parent-child interaction patterns.

The correct response is Option D: Marital and parent-child interaction patterns.

Falicov (2012) has developed a multilevel model for prevention and intervention with transnational families, integrating three contexts in risk and resilience: the relational level, the community level, and the cultural-sociopolitical level. The relational context deals with marital and parent-child interaction patterns that are a product of the migration experience.

The community level addresses the loss of social networks and the reconstitution of new and old community bonds.

The sociopolitical level attends to cultural diversity issues and encounters with prejudice and discrimination that affect adaptation. **(p. 629)**

3.	In divorce and stepfamily formation, what matters most for successful adaptation?

A. Not having joint custody even when parents can cooperate.
B. Parents staying together in an unhappy marriage rather than getting a divorce.
C. The quality of relationships with parents and between parents.
D. Receiving divorce mediation and collaborative counseling.

The correct response is Option C: The quality of relationships with parents and between parents.

What matters most for successful adaptation in the process of divorce and stepfamily formation is the quality of relationships with parents and between parents before and after divorce.

Joint custody works well when parents cooperate in decision-making, child contact, financial support, and shared responsibilities.

Although grown children may have painful memories of the divorce, most have no greater difficulty developing committed intimate relationships than those whose parents stayed unhappily married.

Mediation and collaborative or cooperative divorce counseling are recommended. However, this is not considered to be the most influential for the family's adaptation. **(p. 628)**

4.	Which of these situations is an example of disenfranchised loss?

A. Homicide.
B. Miscarriage.

C. Dementia.

D. Fatal accident.

The correct response is Option B: Miscarriage.

The nature and circumstances of loss can complicate bereavement, increasing the risk of child and family dysfunction. Disenfranchised losses, such as socially unacknowledged losses (e.g., miscarriages, death of a pet) or stigmatized deaths (as with HIV/AIDS or suicide) can lead to secrecy, guilt, and estrangement.

Violent deaths, such as fatal accidents, homicide, or suicide, can generate lingering anger, guilt, remorse, and forgiveness issues.

Ambiguous loss occurs when there is a lack of clarity about the fate of a missing loved one or when there is psychological and relational loss of a loved one who is still alive, as in dementia. **(pp. 625–626)**

5.   A 12-year-old girl recently lost her mother in a fatal car accident. The girl lives with her father, and the rest of the extended family lives out of state. As the mental health clinician for this family, which of the following should you recommend to minimize long-term complications associated with the loss of the mother?

A. Mobilize the kin network.

B. Minimize the meaning of loss.

C. Suggest that the surviving parent remarry soon.

D. Encourage the child to suppress her grief to support her father.

The correct response is Option A: Mobilize the kin network.

Children who lose a parent are at risk for long-term complications such as difficulty forming intimate attachments or catastrophic fears of separation and abandonment. Therefore, it is important to mobilize the kin network to provide support, structure, and reassurance that children will be cared for and not suffer further loss.

In the death of a parent, adolescents may minimize the meaning of loss, but minimization is not a helpful phenomenon in reducing long-term complications.

Mourning is important in tragic deaths. Financial and childrearing demands can interfere with a surviving parent's mourning processes. Mourning can also be blocked if children suppress their grief to support the parent or if well-meaning relatives push for premature closure and precipitous replacement of a spouse or parent. **(p. 626)**

Reference

Falicov CJ: Immigrant family processes: a multidimensional framework, in Normal Family Processes, 4th Edition. Edited by Walsh F. New York, Guilford, 2012, pp 297–323

C H A P T E R   3 1

Legal and Ethical Issues

Tapan Parikh, M.D., M.P.H.
Mina K. Dulcan, M.D.

1. Which of the following is true regarding the ethical principle of confidentiality when treating minors?

   A. The confidential information disclosed by a minor must be disclosed to a parent or guardian, and the minor should be informed of this.
   B. The confidential information disclosed by a minor must be disclosed to a parent or guardian; however, the minor does not need to be informed of this.
   C. The clinician should articulate the issues involved in confidentiality and informed consent as the treatment progresses. These are not important in the initial phase of treatment when rapport is still being built.
   D. This principle obligates the clinician to hold in confidence communications with the patient, even if a minor.

The correct response is Option D: This principle obligates the clinician to hold in confidence communications with the patient, even if a minor.

The ethical principle of confidentiality is considered the cornerstone for building trust and honest communication in the physician-patient relationship. This principle obligates the clinician to hold in confidence communications with the patient; even if a minor, the patient is the holder of the right to confidentiality and must give consent for the release of that information. However, as with all children under the legal age, the parents or legal guardian must give the legal consent for evaluation and treatment, except when there are specific statutory exceptions. Such exemptions include mandatory reporting of child abuse, emancipated minors, or situations in which a child is an imminent danger to self or others. In clinical practice with children and parent(s), the clinician should articulate the issues involved in confidentiality and informed consent with both the child and the parent(s) or legal guardian during the beginning of the evaluation process, taking into account the child's level of understanding and ability to assent. **(pp. 639–640)**

2.   Which of the following is *not* in line with the regulatory guidance regarding the Health Insurance Portability and Accountability Act (HIPAA) from the U.S. Department of Health and Human Services?

A. Unless a competent patient objects, the psychiatrist and other clinicians can speak with other family members assisting in the patient's treatment.
B. When psychiatric disorder or substance abuse impairs a patient's capacities, mental health professionals may share patient-related information in the patient's best interest.
C. Although the laws can vary from state to state, in no state can the laws regarding mental health confidentiality be stricter than the HIPAA regulations.
D. Certain disclosures are permissible when patients present a serious and imminent threat to themselves or others.

The correct response is Option C: Although the laws can vary from state to state, in no state can the laws regarding mental health confidentiality be stricter than the HIPAA regulations.

Recent subregulatory guidance regarding HIPAA from the U.S. Department of Health and Human Services covers the rules governing disclosures to parents of minor patients, including the following:

• Unless a competent patient objects, the psychiatrist and other clinicians can speak with other family members who are assisting in the patient's treatment.
• When psychiatric disorder or substance abuse impairs a patient's capacities, mental health professionals can share patient-related information in the patient's best interest.
• Certain disclosures are permissible when patients present a serious and imminent threat to themselves or others.

In some states, however, the laws regarding mental health confidentiality are stricter than the HIPAA regulations. **(p. 641)**

3.   Which of the following is *not* true regarding emancipated minors?

A. Emancipated minors are generally older than age 15 years, living away from parents, and economically self-sufficient.
B. Minors living with extended families or foster families are considered emancipated.
C. Married minors are considered emancipated.
D. Minors on active duty in the U.S. armed services are considered emancipated.

The correct response is Option B: Minors living with extended families or foster families are considered emancipated.

Emancipated minors can consent to their own treatment. This group generally includes minors who are older than age 15 years, living away from parents, and economically self-sufficient; married minors; minors on active duty in the U.S. armed services; and minors who have been emancipated through a specific court order. Courts can also determine that a minor is "mature" and able to appreciate the nature, extent, and consequences of medical treatment. Minors living with extended or foster families are not considered emancipated. **(p. 641)**

4.   Which of the following is not part of the four elements of a professional negligence claim?

   A. Beneficence.
   B. Duty.
   C. Dereliction.
   D. Damages.

The correct response is Option A: Beneficence.

Child psychiatrists have become increasingly subject to malpractice suits in the past few decades. These suits are based on principles of tort law or wrongful civil behavior, in which the practitioner may be liable for the unintended consequences of alleged harm or injury to the patient or to a third party that could have or should have been prevented by the practitioner's action. The four elements of a claim of professional negligence are 1) duty—a duty of care was owed to the patient by the physician; 2) dereliction—the duty of care was breached; 3) damages—the patient experienced actual damage due to the breach of duty; and 4) direct causation—the dereliction was the direct cause of the damages.

   Beneficence is a term that expands the "do no harm" concept to include acting in the patient's best interests and minimizing risks and maximizing benefits in professional judgments and relationships; this is not an element of a claim of professional negligence. **(pp. 639, 642)**

5.   Which of the following accurately describes standards of evidence used in the legal system?

   A. The standard of a preponderance of the evidence (i.e., more likely than not) cannot be used in most civil proceedings.
   B. The highest standard of proof, "beyond a reasonable doubt," is required in cases where deprivation of fundamental rights or liberty is at stake, such as termination of parental rights.
   C. The intermediate standard of "clear and convincing evidence" is needed in juvenile court and delinquency proceedings.
   D. The highest standard of proof, "beyond a reasonable doubt," is used in criminal proceedings.

The correct response is Option D: The highest standard of proof, "beyond a reasonable doubt," is used in criminal proceedings.

The *standard of proof* is the level of certainty required for a certain judicial outcome, and it varies depending on the type of legal proceeding. For example, the standard of a preponderance of the evidence (i.e., more likely than not) is used in most civil proceedings.

The intermediate standard of "clear and convincing evidence" is required in cases where a deprivation of fundamental rights or liberty is at stake, such as termination of parental rights.

The highest standard of proof, "beyond a reasonable doubt," is used in criminal proceedings as well as juvenile court and delinquency proceedings. **(pp. 642–643)**

6.   Child psychiatrists are increasingly being called on to testify as experts in various legal proceedings. Which of the following is true when the child and adolescent psychiatrist acts as an expert witness?

A.   The psychiatrist's opinion as an expert witness may ultimately result in harm to the child.
B.   Although a child psychiatrist who is acting as an expert witness does not usually function in a doctor-patient relationship in the case, some exceptions exist.
C.   When a psychiatrist is serving as an expert witness, the client is usually a parent or guardian.
D.   As an expert witness, the child psychiatrist writes a report, provides depositions, and/or testifies in court and may provide treatment recommendations to the patient's treating psychiatrist.

The correct response is Option A: The psychiatrist's opinion as an expert witness may ultimately result in harm to the child.

The role of an expert witness is distinguished from the role of treating clinician by the absence of a doctor-patient relationship; there are generally no exceptions to this. The psychiatrist's opinion may even ultimately result in harm to the child. For example, the child may be waived to an adult court or taken away from the parents in a dependency hearing.

As expert witnesses, child psychiatrists draw on their specific body of knowledge to form an opinion about a legal issue, not an ethical issue. No treatment is rendered or recommended, and the usual medical, legal, and ethical principles regarding interactions between physicians and patients do not apply. The psychiatrist's client is the attorney or the court who is hiring the psychiatrist to render an expert opinion.

Acting as an expert witness, the psychiatrist is typically asked to read legal documents; conduct interviews; and then write a report, provide depositions, and/or testify in court. As an expert witness, child psychiatrists do not provide treatment recommendations to the patients, families, or treating psychiatrists. **(p. 644)**

7.   Which of the following is *not* an example of competence criteria that allow children to provide testimony?

A. The capacity to register an event.
B. The ability to accurately recall and recount the event.
C. The capacity to communicate on the basis of suggestibility.
D. The ability to distinguish truth from falsehood.

The correct response is Option C: The capacity to communicate on the basis of suggestibility.

Because sexual abuse allegations frequently lack physical evidence, the child's testimony in these cases is often critical. A body of information has been developed regarding children's competency, memory, suggestibility, and credibility. A child's competency to act as a witness refers to the ability to testify in court in a reliable and meaningful manner. Competence is determined by four criteria: the capacity to register an event, the ability to recall and recount the event accurately, the ability to distinguish truth from falsehood, and the capacity to communicate on the basis of personal knowledge of the facts. The last criterion refers to communication that is based on personal knowledge and facts and not based on suggestibility, which is a concern that can lead to deviation from the facts in this age group. The literature shows that children are highly suggestible, with preschool-age children being more suggestible than older children or adults. **(p. 647)**

C H A P T E R   3 2

Telemental Health and e-Mental Health Applications With Children and Adolescents

Ewa Bieber, M.D.

1.   Which of the following is a requirement under the Ryan Haight Online Pharmacy Consumer Protection Act of 2008?

A. Pharmacies must keep a record of medications prescribed during telemental health visits.
B. Controlled substances may not be prescribed during telemental health visits.
C. Physicians must complete one in-person evaluation of the patient prior to prescribing a controlled substance.
D. Patients using telemental health visits must fill prescriptions at online pharmacies.

The correct response is Option C: Physicians must complete one in-person evaluation of the patient prior to prescribing a controlled substance.

The Ryan Haight Online Pharmacy Consumer Protection Act of 2008 (Pub. L. No. 110-425; www.gpo.gov/fdsys/pkg/PLAW-110publ425/html/PLAW-110publ425.htm) was designed to expunge illegitimate online pharmacies that dispensed controlled substances without physician oversight, but it also inadvertently placed certain restrictions around the practice of prescribing by means of the internet. Although the act specifies that telemedicine is an exception, it technically requires that physicians conduct at least one in-person evaluation of the patient prior to prescribing a controlled substance. Controlled substances may then be prescribed during telemental health visits. The act does not require pharmacies to keep records of medications prescribed during telemental health visits, nor does it require patients to use online pharmacies. **(p. 657)**

2. Through which of the following does the Centers for Medicare and Medicaid Services (CMS) define telemedicine as delivering health care services?

    A. A secure phone line.
    B. A real-time interactive conferencing system with audio.
    C. A real-time interactive videoconferencing system with both audio and video.
    D. A specific videoconferencing system licensed by the CMS.

    The correct response is Option C: A real-time interactive videoconferencing system with both audio and video.

    The CMS refer to telemedicine as the delivery of health care services via real-time interactive videoconferencing that includes *both* audio and video components (Centers for Medicare and Medicaid Services 2020). CMS does not license or specify which videoconferencing system should be used. **(p. 653)**

3. Which of the following is *not* necessary during a telemental health visit?

    A. Modern, well-functioning equipment.
    B. Encrypted software.
    C. Consistent high-speed connectivity.
    D. The patient and the clinician must both be at a clinical site.

    The correct response is Option D: The patient and the clinician must both be at a clinical site.

    Telemental health visits allow patients to be seen in nonclinical settings, such as home or school. Both the teleclinician's site and the patient's site must have access to 1) modern, well-functioning equipment, including camera, monitor, microphone, and speakers; 2) encrypted software; 3) secure clinical space for the equipment; and 4) consistent high-speed connectivity. **(p. 658)**

4. Which of the following is true regarding the documentation of a telemental health visit?

    A. A clear indication that the clinical visit was conducted through videoconferencing is a must, but it is not necessary to document the patient's and clinician's locations.
    B. The name of the videoconferencing system used must be documented.

C. The patient's and clinician's locations during the visit need to be documented, but documenting a clear indication that the clinical visit was conducted through videoconferencing is optional.
D. A clear indication that the clinical visit was conducted through videoconferencing and the locations of the patient and the clinician during the visit need to be documented.

The correct response is Option D: A clear indication that the clinical visit was conducted through videoconferencing and the locations of the patient and the clinician during the visit need to be documented.

Telemental health involves some unique issues in documentation. The documentation must clearly indicate that the clinical visit was conducted through videoconferencing, as well as provide the locations of the patient and clinician during the session. It does not require the name of the videoconference system used. **(p. 667)**

5.   Which of the following can be used to improve audio privacy during telemental health visits?

A. Whispering.
B. Encouraging patients to type sensitive information in the chat feature.
C. Adding pillows to couches, curtains on windows, or tapestries on walls.
D. Placing a white noise machine next to the videoconferencing equipment's speakers.

The correct response is Option C: Adding pillows to couches, curtains on windows, or tapestries on walls.

Audio privacy may be the largest obstacle to privacy during telemedicine visits. If the patient site is a clinical examination room, it would already have been soundproofed. However, the videoconferencing equipment often is set up in a conference room, private office, or home with inadequate soundproofing. Placing pillows on couches, curtains on windows, and/or tapestries on walls to absorb sound aids in improving audio privacy. Microphones may alter a person's voice, so speaking clearly, with normal volume and enunciation, is encouraged. Individual sessions, and some parent-child sessions, may be conducted away from other family members in a bedroom or office or on a porch. Patients should not be encouraged to share sensitive information if audio privacy is not established. A white noise machine may be placed outside the room or by the door but would interfere with the ability to hear if placed next to the speakers. The patients may prefer not to type sensitive information in the chat feature, which may not be confidential anyway. Additionally, the chat feature does not address the question of audio privacy improvement. Further methods for improving audio privacy and minimizing background noise are listed in Tables 32–2 and 32–3. **(pp. 661–662)**

6. What contract between the health care entity and the internet vendor is required for telemedicine visits?

    A. The online telemedicine payment contract.
    B. The business associate agreement (BAA).
    C. The Health Insurance Portability and Accountability Act contract for telemedicine (HIPAA-CT).
    D. The managed care agreement.

    The correct response is Option B: The business associate agreement (BAA).

    A HIPAA-covered entity is typically a health care provider, health plan, or health care clearinghouse that conducts transactions electronically. Under HIPAA, a vendor of a HIPAA-covered entity that needs to be provided with protected health information (PHI) to perform duties on behalf of the covered entity is called a business associate. A vendor is also classed as a business associate if electronic PHI (ePHI) passes through its system. The internet vendor should have signed a business associate agreement, a contract to ensure the security of patients' PHI (see www.hipaajournal.com/hipaa-business-associate-agreement). The covered entity must obtain a signed business associate agreement before allowing a business associate to come into contact with PHI or ePHI. **(pp. 656–657)**

Reference

Centers for Medicare and Medicaid Services: Telemedicine. Baltimore, MD, Centers for Medicare and Medicaid Services, 2020. Available at: www.medicaid.gov/medicaid/benefits/telemedicine/index.html. Accessed March 8, 2020.

CHAPTER 33

Principles of Psychopharmacology

Esther S. Lee, M.D.

Robert L. Findling, M.D., M.B.A.

1.   Interviewing children can be more challenging compared with older adolescents
      or adults for all of the following reasons *except*

      A. Developmental variability in psychological and cognitive characteristics.
      B. Relative limitations in verbal abilities.
      C. More comfort and experience in recognizing emotions and feelings.
      D. Difficulty accurately estimating time increments.

      **The correct response is Option C: More comfort and experience in recognizing
      emotions and feelings.**

      One of the challenges in interviewing younger patients is that they have less ex-
      perience in recognizing their emotions and feelings than do older youth or adults.
      Other challenges in interviewing younger patients may include developmental
      variability in psychological and cognitive characteristics, relatively limited verbal
      abilities, and difficulty accurately estimating time increments. **(p. 680)**

2.   Preemptive cardiovascular risk stratification with a baseline electrocardiogram
      (ECG) may be important when considering higher-risk psychotropic medica-
      tions, including all of the following *except*

      A. Lithium.
      B. First-generation antipsychotics.
      C. Carbamazepine.
      D. Tricyclic antidepressants.

The correct response is Option C: Carbamazepine.

It is suggested that a complete blood count, including platelets, should be obtained as a baseline before treatment with carbamazepine, but an ECG is not routinely recommended. Higher-risk medications that may require a baseline ECG include α_2-adrenergic receptor agonists (such as clonidine or guanfacine), first-generation antipsychotics (especially pimozide), atypical antipsychotics (such as clozapine and ziprasidone), tricyclic antidepressants, lithium, and stimulants. **(p. 683)**

3.   Pharmacokinetic differences between children and adults include all of the following *except*

   A. When adjusted for body weight, children may have proportionally more liver tissue than adults.
   B. Children may have proportionally more extracellular and total-body water than adults.
   C. Children may have proportionally less fat tissue than adults.
   D. Children may have lower glomerular filtration rates than adults when adjusted for body weight.

The correct response is Option D: Children may have lower glomerular filtration rates than adults when adjusted for body weight.

Children may have *higher* glomerular filtration rates than adults when adjusted for body weight, possibly resulting in more rapid excretion of drugs that use renal pathways. The following pharmacokinetic understandings are true: 1) Children may have proportionally more liver tissue than adults when adjusted for body weight. 2) Children may have proportionally more extracellular and total-body water than adults. 3) Children may have proportionally less fat tissue than adults. **(p. 687)**

4.   Which of the following federal legislative acts first gave pharmaceutical companies greater financial incentives to voluntarily conduct clinical trials of medications in children and adolescents?

   A. The Pediatric Research Equity Act (PREA).
   B. The U.S. Food and Drug Administration Modernization Act of 1997 (FDAMA).
   C. The Best Pharmaceuticals for Children Act (BPCA).
   D. The U.S. Food and Drug Administration Safety and Innovation Act.

The correct response is Option B: The U.S. Food and Drug Administration Modernization Act of 1997 (FDAMA).

In 1997, FDAMA created financial incentives for pediatric clinical trials. The BPCA renewed these incentives in 2002, and the PREA in 2003 authorized the FDA to require pediatric studies of drugs in development if those drugs had the potential for use in the young. The U.S. Food and Drug Administration Safety and

Innovation Act of 2012 made BPCA and PREA permanent, in addition to empowering the FDA to ensure that the requirements were met by manufacturers in a timely manner. **(p. 689)**

5. All of the following reasons may contribute to treatment nonadherence to psychopharmacological treatment *except*

    A. An authoritative communication style used by the clinician.
    B. The emergence of adverse drug effects.
    C. The social stigma associated with mental illness.
    D. Pressure from family expectations or cultural beliefs.

    The correct response is Option A: An authoritative communication style used by the clinician.

    The authoritative communication style, which involves presenting treatment options and asking the family to choose one, often develops positive rapport and a strong therapeutic alliance with the patient and family. This, in turn, frequently increases confidence in both the provider and the selected treatment option. Reasons for nonadherence may include the perception that the drug is not effective, the emergence of adverse drug effects, misperceived expectations about the possible effects of psychotropic medications, peer pressure in the form of teasing or ridicule, the social stigma associated with mental illness, pressure from family expectations or cultural beliefs, or the patient's resistance to following directions from parents and other adults. **(pp. 686, 692–693)**

CHAPTER 34

Medications Used for ADHD

Ronald Steingard, M.D.

Mark A. Stein, Ph.D.

John S. Markowitz, Pharm.D.

1. Which of the following options includes medications approved by the FDA for the treatment of ADHD?

    A. Methylphenidate, amphetamine, and bupropion.
    B. Guanfacine, amphetamine, and atomoxetine.
    C. Amphetamine, bupropion, and modafinil.
    D. Guanfacine, amphetamine, and modafinil.

    The correct response is Option B: Guanfacine, amphetamine, and atomoxetine.

    The three stimulants that are FDA approved for ADHD are methylphenidate, amphetamine, and methamphetamine (very rarely used). Three nonstimulant compounds that are FDA approved for ADHD include atomoxetine, clonidine, and guanfacine. Modafinil and bupropion are often used off-label and have some research support but have not received approval from the FDA for this indication. **(p. 696)**

2. Which of the following is true regarding treatment options for ADHD?

    A. Biological markers can be used to predict individual responses to ADHD treatments.
    B. Given the tolerability of stimulant medications, they can be started at the maximum recommended dose.

C. Atomoxetine has been associated with initial weight loss.

D. Bupropion, used off-label for ADHD, was originally developed as an antipsychotic.

The correct response is Option C: Atomoxetine has been associated with initial weight loss.

Atomoxetine, a selective noradrenergic reuptake inhibitor approved by the FDA in 2002 for use in treating ADHD in children and adults, has been associated with initial weight loss.

Biological markers have not yet been shown to predict individual response to different pharmacotherapies.

It is not advised to initiate treatment with stimulants at the maximum allowed dose. Rather, given the marked interindividual variability, it is best to introduce the medication at a low dose and titrate the dose stepwise.

Bupropion is an aminoketone originally developed as an antidepressant and later approved for smoking cessation. **(pp. 703, 717)**

3. Which of the following stimulant formulations has both a rapid onset of action and a brief duration of response?

A. Concerta.

B. Jornay PM.

C. Evekeo.

D. Mydayis.

The correct response is Option C: Evekeo.

Evekeo is the only immediate-release (brief-duration) stimulant in this list. Jornay PM, Concerta, and Mydayis are all extended-release formulations. Jornay PM has a delayed onset of response. **(pp. 706–710, Tables 34–3 to 34–5)**

4. All of the following statements are true for the optimal treatment of ADHD with medication *except*

A. Individualized dose titration is important.

B. Routine monitoring using standard measures is necessary.

C. Ongoing assessments should include observing for any side effects.

D. Vital signs monitoring at baseline is necessary, but there is no need to monitor routinely.

The correct response is Option D: Vital signs monitoring at baseline is necessary, but there is no need to monitor routinely.

Optimal treatment should include vital signs monitoring at baseline as well as during follow-up visits as part of ongoing monitoring. Individualized dose titration is important because individuals may respond differently to a particular dose. Routine monitoring using standard measures is necessary. These routine and ongoing assessments should include observation for any side effects. **(p. 723)**

5. Which of the following statements is true regarding treatment adherence for ADHD in adolescents?

   A. Treatment adherence tends not to be an issue with standard treatment.
   B. Treatment adherence appears to be unrelated to concerns about stigma.
   C. Treatment adherence can be made worse by including the patient in treatment decisions.
   D. Treatment adherence can be improved with ongoing psychoeducation, medication adjustments, and shared decision-making.

   The correct response is Option D: Treatment adherence can be improved with ongoing psychoeducation, medication adjustments, and shared decision-making.

   Treatment adherence is often an issue in adolescents, and it can be improved with ongoing psychoeducation, medication adjustments, and shared decision-making. Issues related to treatment compliance are common in adolescents and may be related to the stigma associated with diagnosis and treatment. Failure to listen to the adolescent's concerns or to involve the adolescent in treatment decisions can increase the likelihood of treatment nonadherence. Ongoing psychoeducation about the disorder and available treatments, medication adjustment in response to the patient's stated concerns, and shared decision-making that includes the adolescent may decrease the risk of nonadherence. **(pp. 697, 723)**

6. Which of the following is true regarding amphetamines?

   A. Amphetamines decrease the synaptic availability of dopamine and norepinephrine.
   B. Amphetamines hasten the reuptake of catecholamines from the synaptic cleft.
   C. Amphetamines increase the production of dopamine and norepinephrine.
   D. Amphetamines displace monoamines from intraneuronal storage vesicles.

   The correct response is Option D: Amphetamines displace monoamines from intraneuronal storage vesicles.

   Amphetamine increases dopamine's and norepinephrine's availability, not production, by blocking the reuptake of catecholamines from the synaptic cleft. In addition, amphetamines also enter the presynaptic cell and displace monoamines from storage vesicles, resulting in a reversal of the flow of the reuptake pump, further increasing the availability of all monoamines (including serotonin) in the synaptic cleft. **(p. 701)**

7. Cardiovascular effects of α_2-adrenergic receptor agonists include which of the following?

A. Increased blood pressure.
B. Decreased electrocardiogram PR interval.
C. Decreased heart rate.
D. Decreased ECG QTcF interval.

The correct response is Option C: Decreased heart rate.

α_2-Adrenergic receptor agonists were originally developed as antihypertensives, and they decrease blood pressure and heart rate and increase PR interval and QTcF interval, as seen on the ECG. Heart rate and blood pressure should be monitored during treatment. Changes in heart rate and blood pressure may be most pronounced at the beginning of treatment and can lessen as treatment continues. Caution should be exercised in individuals with a history of preexisting hypotension, atrioventricular block, bradycardia, or known cardiovascular disease. In these individuals, a consultation with a pediatric cardiologist before starting treatment is warranted. **(p. 712)**

CHAPTER 35

Antidepressants

Graham J. Emslie, M.D.

Jessica M. Jones, M.A.

Laura A. Stone, M.D.

1. Which of the following medications is *not* contraindicated in a patient taking a selective serotonin reuptake inhibitor (SSRI)?

    A. Pimozide.
    B. Selegiline.
    C. Trifluoperazine.
    D. Linezolid.

    The correct response is Option C: Trifluoperazine.

    Pimozide is contraindicated in combination with SSRIs because of the risk of QT prolongation. The concomitant use of SSRIs and monoamine oxidase inhibitors (MAOIs) is contraindicated because of the risk of serotonin syndrome. MAOIs include selegiline, linezolid, intravenous methylene blue, phenelzine, isocarboxazid, and tranylcypromine. MAOIs modulate the concentration of monoamines in the CNS by inhibiting either MAO-A or MAO-B isoforms. SSRIs should not be taken with an MAOI or within 2 weeks after MAOI discontinuation because this combination may lead to severe serotonin syndrome. **(pp. 732, 750)**

2. When considering the pharmacodynamics of antidepressants, what is unique about sertraline?

    A. It is the only SSRI with an affinity for dopamine receptors.
    B. At low dosages, it is primarily an SSRI. At higher dosages, it also acts as a norepinephrine reuptake inhibitor.

C. It is the most potent serotonin and norepinephrine reuptake inhibitor among the SSRIs.
D. It inhibits the reuptake of norepinephrine and dopamine.

The correct response is Option A: It is the only SSRI with an affinity for dopamine receptors.

Sertraline is the only SSRI with an affinity for dopamine receptors.

Duloxetine and venlafaxine act as SSRIs at lower dosages and as selective serotonin-norepinephrine reuptake inhibitors (SSNRIs) at higher dosages.

Paroxetine hydrochloride is structurally unrelated to other antidepressants. Paroxetine is the SSRI with the most potent serotonin and norepinephrine reuptake inhibition. Sertraline is the second-most potent SSRI (after paroxetine) and the only SSRI with an affinity for dopamine receptors.

Bupropion inhibits the reuptake of norepinephrine and dopamine and is classified as a norepinephrine and dopamine reuptake inhibitor. **(pp. 740–741, 747, 749, 751)**

3.   Which atypical antidepressant (non-SSRI) has received approval from the FDA for use in youth?

A. Mirtazapine.
B. Bupropion.
C. Trazodone.
D. Duloxetine.

The correct response is Option D: Duloxetine.

Duloxetine has an FDA-approved indication for the treatment of generalized anxiety disorder in youth ages 7–17 years. Mirtazapine, bupropion, and trazodone have FDA-approved indications only in adults. **(pp. 743, Table 35–4; 749)**

4.   Which two antidepressants have received approval from the FDA for the treatment of depression in adolescents?

A. Citalopram and escitalopram.
B. Escitalopram and fluoxetine.
C. Fluoxetine and fluvoxamine.
D. Paroxetine and sertraline.

The correct response is Option B: Escitalopram and fluoxetine.

Escitalopram has an FDA-approved indication for the treatment of depression in adolescents (ages 12 years and up), and fluoxetine has an FDA-approved indication for the treatment of depression in children and adolescents (ages 8 years and up). Citalopram, paroxetine, and sertraline have FDA-approved indications for the treatment of depression in adults only. Fluvoxamine has an FDA-approved indication in adolescents only for the treatment of OCD. **(pp. 735, 738)**

5. Which SSRI that may be used for the treatment of OCD in youth is more likely to cause discontinuation symptoms due to its short half-life?

   A. Fluoxetine.
   B. Fluvoxamine.
   C. Paroxetine.
   D. Sertraline.

The correct response is Option C: Paroxetine.

Fluoxetine, fluvoxamine, paroxetine, and sertraline all have had positive randomized controlled trials in youth with OCD. Paroxetine's side effects are similar to those of other SSRIs. Because of paroxetine's short half-life, its discontinuation symptoms are thought to be more severe than those of other SSRIs. In randomized controlled trials of paroxetine in pediatric major depressive disorder and OCD, 10% of the paroxetine-treated patients withdrew early because of adverse events. **(p. 740)**

6. Which of the following atypical antidepressants is a nonselective N-methyl-D-aspartate (NMDA) antagonist?

   A. Bupropion.
   B. Ketamine.
   C. Levomilnacipran.
   D. Vortioxetine.

The correct response is Option B: Ketamine.

Unlike conventional antidepressants, which target modulatory monoaminergic neurotransmitters (serotonin, norepinephrine, and dopamine), ketamine is a nonselective, noncompetitive NMDA antagonist. Bupropion is a norepinephrine-dopamine reuptake inhibitor. Levomilnacipran is an SSNRI. Vortioxetine is a serotonin modulator and stimulator. **(p. 753)**

7. When does antidepressant-induced activation typically emerge?

   A. On discontinuation of the medication.
   B. When the maximum recommended dosage is exceeded.
   C. On achieving a steady state of medication.
   D. Early in treatment or following a dosage increase.

The correct response is Option D: Early in treatment or following a dosage increase.

It is important to recognize both antidepressant-induced activation and antidepressant-induced mania. Antidepressant-induced activation, characterized by a state of hyperarousal that may include disinhibition, impulsivity, insomnia, irritability, and restlessness, most often emerges early in treatment or following a dosage increase. This effect has been characterized best in the use of SSRIs and SSNRIs. Antidepressant-induced mania has not been fully studied in youth, although one review article estimated a 2% risk in pediatric patients (Cheung et al. 2005). **(p. 731)**

Reference

Cheung AH, Emslie GJ, Mayes TL: Review of the efficacy and safety of antidepressants in youth depression. J Child Psychol Psychiatry 46(7):735–754, 2005 15972068

CHAPTER 36

Mood Stabilizers

Courtney Heim, D.O.

1.   Which of the following is true regarding lithium treatment for bipolar disorder?

A. Serious neurological symptoms such as seizures, coma, and death can occur when lithium level is above 2 mEq/L.
B. Lithium is FDA approved for the treatment of acute manic and mixed states in patients ages 7 years and older as monotherapy and maintenance treatment of bipolar I disorder.
C. Baseline electrocardiogram (ECG) is not necessary with lithium treatment initiation.
D. Diabetes insipidus is an irreversible adverse effect following lithium use.

The correct response is Option B: Lithium is FDA approved for the treatment of acute manic and mixed states in patients ages 7 years and older as monotherapy and maintenance treatment of bipolar I disorder.

Lithium is the only mood stabilizer indicated by the FDA for the treatment of acute manic and mixed states in patients ages 7 years and older as monotherapy and maintenance treatment of bipolar I disorder.

Lithium has a very narrow therapeutic window (0.8–1.2 mEq/L), and patients may develop signs of lithium toxicity when this window is exceeded. The signs of lithium toxicity include nausea, vomiting, slurred speech, and dyscoordination. In addition, with blood levels above 3.0 mEq/L, patients may develop more serious neurological symptoms, including seizures, coma, and death.

Lithium occasionally may affect cardiac conduction, and therefore a baseline ECG should be obtained, and, ideally, another ECG is recommended once a therapeutic lithium level has been reached.

Diabetes insipidus is reversible if lithium is discontinued. **(pp. 763–765)**

2.   A 15-year-old male adolescent with a past psychiatric history of bipolar disorder is seen in the clinic for follow-up. His mood has been stable on lamotrigine for years. However, he was recently hospitalized because of increasingly severe aggression, and another medication was prescribed to target the aggression. The lamotrigine dosage was unchanged when this new medication was added. Unfortunately, the patient developed erythematous desquamative lesions all over his body, including severe oral ulcers. What is the most likely medication that was started during his hospitalization?

A. Quetiapine.
B. Amitriptyline.
C. Lithium.
D. Valproate.

The correct response is Option D: Valproate.

In children and adolescents, valproate may be effective in the treatment of aggression. However, valproate may increase the levels of medications such as phenobarbital, carbamazepine, phenytoin, tricyclics, and lamotrigine. Therefore, when valproate was added for this patient's aggression, it likely inhibited the clearance of lamotrigine, putting him at a higher risk for developing Stevens-Johnson syndrome (SJS) and toxic epidermal necrolysis (TEN). The dosage of lamotrigine should be reduced when it is coadministered with valproate because of this drug interaction potential. Quetiapine, amitriptyline, and lithium have no effect on the metabolism of lamotrigine. **(p. 769)**

3.   Which medication would be contraindicated in a person with HLA-B gene variant *HLA-B*1502*?

A. Lithium.
B. Lamotrigine.
C. Carbamazepine.
D. Gabapentin.

The correct response is Option C: Carbamazepine.

If the patient is of broad Asian ancestry, there is a strong association between the risk of developing SJS or TEN with carbamazepine treatment and an inherited variant of the HLA-B gene *HLA-B*1502*. *HLA-B*1502* is largely absent in individuals not of Asian origin (e.g., whites, African Americans, Hispanics, American Indians). Because of this risk, all patients of Asian ancestry should undergo HLA typing before starting carbamazepine. There is no such risk with the other options. **(p. 771)**

4.   A 17-year-old female adolescent was started on lamotrigine as a maintenance medication to prevent future mood episodes. A new medication was added, and

shortly afterward, she had a reoccurrence of depressive symptoms. What medication was likely added?

A. Valproate.
B. Carbamazepine.
C. Lithium.
D. Topiramate.

The correct response is Option B: Carbamazepine.

Adding carbamazepine to lamotrigine decreases lamotrigine blood levels by 50%, likely leading to clinical destabilization in this case with reemergence of mood symptoms. Carbamazepine has many clinically significant drug interactions because it stimulates the hepatic cytochrome P450 isoenzyme system. Carbamazepine decreases lithium clearance, increasing the risk of lithium toxicity. Carbamazepine may also decrease the levels of the following medications: oral contraceptives, clonazepam, glucocorticoids, phenobarbital, primidone, phenytoin, tricyclics, valproate, and many of the atypical antipsychotics. **(pp. 771–772)**

5.   Oxcarbazepine is structurally related to carbamazepine—that is, oxcarbazepine is the 10-keto analogue of carbamazepine. Which of the following is true regarding differences between clinical use of carbamazepine and oxcarbazepine?

A. Both carbamazepine and oxcarbazepine carry FDA-approved indications for acute manic and mixed episodes in bipolar I disorder in adults.
B. Carbamazepine is indicated by the FDA for the treatment of partial seizures but not generalized tonic seizures, and the same is true for oxcarbazepine.
C. Although oxcarbazepine has an FDA indication for the treatment of certain mood episodes in adults with bipolar I disorder, carbamazepine does not have any evidence base for the treatment of bipolar disorder.
D. Although carbamazepine has an FDA indication for the treatment of certain mood episodes in adults with bipolar I disorder, oxcarbazepine does not have any evidence base for the treatment of bipolar disorder.

The correct response is option D: Although carbamazepine has an FDA indication for the treatment of certain mood episodes in adults with bipolar I disorder, oxcarbazepine does not have any evidence base for the treatment of bipolar disorder.

Carbamazepine is indicated by the FDA for the treatment of partial seizures with complex symptoms (psychomotor, temporal lobe), generalized tonic seizures (grand mal), mixed seizure patterns, trigeminal neuralgia, and acute manic and mixed episodes in bipolar I disorder in adults. Oxcarbazepine is indicated by the FDA for use as monotherapy or adjunctive therapy in the treatment of partial seizures in adults and as monotherapy in the treatment of partial seizures in children.

No evidence has been found for the efficacy of oxcarbazepine for treating mania, hypomania, or bipolar depression in adults. Oxcarbazepine is not known to be useful for any psychiatric disorders in children and adolescents. **(pp. 770, 772)**

CHAPTER 37

Antipsychotic Medications

Abdullah Bin Mahfodh, M.D.

1. Which of the following is correct regarding cytochrome P450 (CYP) enzymes and the metabolism of antipsychotics?

    A. CYP3A4 is a low-affinity, high-capacity enzyme most relevant in the metabolism of aripiprazole, iloperidone, perphenazine, and risperidone.
    B. CYP2D6 is a high-affinity, low-capacity enzyme most relevant in the metabolism of clozapine and olanzapine.
    C. CYP1A2 is a low-affinity, high-capacity enzyme that is relevant for the clearance of clozapine and, to some degree, olanzapine.
    D. CYP2C19 and 2C9 are relevant only for risperidone clearance.

    The correct response is Option C: CYP1A2 is a low-affinity, high-capacity enzyme that is relevant for the clearance of clozapine and, to some degree, olanzapine.

    The CYP enzymes 3A4, 2D6, and 1A2 are the most important for antipsychotic clearance. CYP3A4 is a low-affinity, high-capacity enzyme, making it relatively immune to saturation unless very potent inhibitors are present. CYP3A4 is relevant mainly for haloperidol, lurasidone, quetiapine, and olanzapine clearance.

    CYP2D6 is a high-affinity, low-capacity enzyme. It is very efficient and not readily inducible, but it can be saturated more easily. Moreover, most known genetic polymorphisms affect CYP2D6. Aripiprazole, iloperidone, perphenazine, and risperidone are cleared predominantly by CYP2D6.

    CYP2C19 and 2C9 are relevant only for clozapine clearance. **(p. 786)**

2.	Which of the following antipsychotics is approved by the FDA for Tourette's disorder in children and adolescents?

	A. Quetiapine.
	B. Olanzapine.
	C. Brexpiprazole.
	D. Aripiprazole.

	The correct response is Option D: Aripiprazole.

	Aripiprazole is FDA approved for the treatment of Tourette's disorder for people ages 6–17 years. Quetiapine is FDA approved for the treatment of bipolar I disorder manic episodes for people ages 10–17 years and schizophrenia for patients ages 13–17 years. Olanzapine is FDA approved for the treatment of bipolar I disorder manic episodes or bipolar I disorder with mixed features, and schizophrenia for people ages 13–17 years. Brexpiprazole did not have any indication for pediatric age groups until recently; however, there is now an FDA-approved indication for treatment of schizophrenia in people ages 13–17 years. Other antipsychotics approved by the FDA for treating Tourette's disorder in the pediatric population are haloperidol and pimozide. **(pp. 787–793, Table 37–1)**

3.	Tardive dyskinesia is less prevalent in youth than in adults, but it can significantly affect the quality of life and should be appropriately addressed immediately. Which of the following is *not* one of the strategies to address tardive dyskinesia?

	A. Add vitamin B_{12}.
	B. Reduce the dosage of antipsychotic medication.
	C. Add vitamin E.
	D. Increase the dosage of antipsychotic medication (masking).

	The correct response is Option A: Add vitamin B_{12}.

	Adding vitamin E, not vitamin B_{12}, is one of the potential strategies to manage tardive dyskinesia. Other possible strategies include reducing the dosage of antipsychotic medication, increasing the dosage of antipsychotic medication (masking), replacing an antipsychotic with a nonantipsychotic when appropriate, and switching to clozapine. **(p. 833, Table 37–9)**

4.	Which of the following is true regarding side effects of antipsychotic medications in children and adolescents?

	A. All antipsychotic medications are associated with a risk of developing myocarditis.
	B. Children and adolescents are less sensitive than adults to extrapyramidal side effects (EPS) associated with first-generation antipsychotics (FGAs) and second-generation antipsychotics (SGAs).

C. Withdrawal dyskinesia rates appear to be higher with SGAs than FGAs.

D. The weight gain potential of SGAs follows roughly the same rank order as in adults, but the magnitude is greater.

The correct response is Option D: The weight gain potential of SGAs follows roughly the same rank order as in adults, but the magnitude is greater.

The weight gain potential of SGAs follows roughly the same rank order as found in adults, but the magnitude is greater. Exceptions may be a greater relative weight gain propensity with risperidone and a greater likelihood of aripiprazole and ziprasidone not being weight-neutral in pediatric patients. Children and adolescents are generally more sensitive than adults to EPS associated with FGAs and SGAs. During FGA treatment, youth are at risk of developing withdrawal dyskinesias. However, unlike in adults, dyskinesias in youth are frequently reversible. Withdrawal dyskinesia rates appear to be lower with SGAs compared with FGAs. However, switching from an antipsychotic with strong dopamine D_2 affinity (risperidone, aripiprazole) to one with less potent affinity (quetiapine, clozapine) may predispose the patient to withdrawal dyskinesia. Only clozapine has been associated with a myocarditis risk, which is greatest early in treatment. Clinical signs of acute myocarditis include palpitations, chest pain, shortness of breath, and syncope. **(pp. 819, 822–823, 825)**

5. When prescribing antipsychotics, adverse effect assessment and monitoring should be proactive, considering developmental norms and thresholds. All of the following should be monitored or assessed routinely in children and adolescents taking antipsychotic medications *except*

    A. Serum fasting blood glucose (or hemoglobin A1C).
    B. Weight and height (calculate BMI percentile and BMI z-score).
    C. Parkinsonism and akathisia.
    D. Serum prolactin.

The correct response is Option D: Serum prolactin.

In the case of hyperprolactinemia, common causes such as hormonal contraception or pregnancy, hypothyroidism, or renal failure need to be ruled out by measuring serum human chorionic gonadotropin, thyroid-stimulating hormone, or creatinine, respectively. Because the effects of subclinical prolactin elevations are unclear, current thinking dictates that prolactin levels be measured only if clinical symptoms develop.

To assess the risk for hyperglycemia and emerging diabetes, fasting blood glucose should be measured at baseline, at 3 months, and every 6 months.

Ideally, weight should be monitored at each clinical visit. Clinically, the most commonly used measures to monitor weight include absolute weight change, percentage weight change (weight change/baseline weight), and change in BMI. Although easily obtained and valid in adults, these measures are useful only for periods of ≤3 months in pediatric patients because they do not account for normal growth. Therefore, age- and sex-adjusted BMI percentiles (used to determine weight category) and BMI z-scores (used for change over time) need to be calculated using growth charts or calculators based on data from the U.S. Centers for Disease Control and Prevention.

Parkinsonian side effects and akathisia should be monitored at baseline, during titration, at 3 months, and annually (more often if abnormalities are noted). **(pp. 828, 830, Table 37–7)**

6.   Which of the following is an example of a primary prevention strategy for youth treated with antipsychotic medications?

A.   Intensifying healthy lifestyle instructions in overweight patients and those with mild baseline metabolic abnormalities, significant weight gain, or beginning metabolic abnormalities during therapy.
B.   Choosing an agent with the lowest likelihood of adverse effects on body composition and metabolic status.
C.   Intensifying weight reduction interventions in patients who are obese or have clinically defined related abnormalities.
D.   Consideration of switching to a lower-risk agent in overweight patients and those with mild baseline metabolic abnormalities, significant weight gain, or beginning metabolic abnormalities during treatment.

The correct response is Option B: Choosing an agent with the lowest likelihood of adverse effects on body composition and metabolic status.

Primary preventive strategies for youth treated with antipsychotics include 1) educating about and maximizing adherence to healthy lifestyle behaviors and 2) choosing an agent with the lowest likelihood of adverse effects on body composition and metabolic status.

Secondary preventive strategies in overweight patients and those with mild baseline metabolic abnormalities, significant weight gain, or beginning metabolic abnormalities during therapy include 1) intensification of healthy lifestyle instructions, 2) consideration of switching to a lower-risk agent, and 3) implementation of a nonpharmacological weight-loss treatment or adjunctive pharmacological intervention that targets normalization or reversal of weight abnormalities.

Tertiary preventive strategies in patients who are obese or have clinically defined related abnormalities (e.g., hyperglycemia, diabetes, dyslipidemia, hypertension) include intensified weight-reduction interventions, attempts at changing to or initiating lower-risk medications for the underlying psychiatric condition, and targeted treatments of these suprathreshold metabolic or endocrine abnormalities, often in conjunction with a subspecialist. **(p. 832)**

7. Antipsychotics may prolong QTc interval. Which of the following is *not* true regarding obtaining a baseline electrocardiogram (ECG)?

A. Obtain an ECG if there is a family history of early sudden death or prolonged QT syndrome.
B. Obtain an ECG if there is a personal history of irregular heartbeat, unexplained tachycardia, or shortness of breath at rest.
C. Because there is a significantly higher risk of QTc prolongation in children and adolescents, an ECG should ideally be obtained at baseline.
D. Obtain an ECG if there is a personal history of dizziness on exertion or syncope.

The correct response is Option C: Because there is a significantly higher risk of QTc prolongation in children and adolescents, an ECG should ideally be obtained at baseline.

In adults, QTc prolongation due to antipsychotics is usually minimal compared with placebo, except for thioridazine. A meta-analysis that evaluated QTc data for nine antipsychotics from 55 prospective studies revealed that aripiprazole decreased QTc interval, whereas risperidone and ziprasidone increased QTc interval (Jensen et al. 2014). QTc prolongation is rare in youth, but the risk is still clinically relevant. Screening for QTc prolongation at baseline is usually indicated when there is a family history of early sudden death or prolonged QT syndrome; a personal history of irregular heartbeat, unexplained tachycardia, or shortness of breath at rest; or a personal history of dizziness on exertion or syncope. **(pp. 824–825)**

Reference

Jensen KG, Juul K, Fink-Jensen A, et al: Corrected QT changes during antipsychotic treatment of children and adolescents: a systematic review and meta-analysis of clinical trials. J Am Acad Child Adolesc Psychiatry 54(1):25–36, 2014 25524787

C H A P T E R   3 8

Individual Psychotherapy

Jonathan Pochyly, Ph.D.

1.   Which of the following terms implies spoken verbal interventions by the therapist commenting on a child's psychological conflicts?

A. Clarification.
B. Interpretations.
C. Reenactment.
D. Mentalization.

The correct response is Option B: Interpretations.

Interpretations are defined as the therapist's bringing together of ideas about the patient's defenses, wishes, conscience, and/or dealings with the world that reveal unconscious mechanisms and thereby make them workable. Anna Freud, Sigmund Freud's daughter, consistently preferred watching and listening to a child and carefully making remarks about the child's conflicts afterward. These spoken verbal interventions by the therapist are called interpretations.

Clarification refers to the therapist's putting new words to something the patient already knows.

Reenactment refers to repetitive behavior (often related to past trauma) that replays a thought, a fear, or an original behavior from the event(s).

Mentalization refers to the ability to reflect on and hold in mind the mental states (feelings, thoughts, beliefs) of oneself and others. **(pp. 848–850)**

2. It is important for a child psychotherapist to include all of the following in any psychotherapy with children *except*

A. A flexible approach to the therapy.
B. Awareness of cultural differences in the child's background.
C. Encouraging a healthy transference of old attitudes to the therapist.
D. Adjustments to meet the child's level of understanding.

The correct response is Option C: Encouraging a healthy transference of old attitudes to the therapist.

Over the years, child psychotherapists have recognized that transference is not as important in the treatment of young children as it is in psychodynamically oriented treatment of adults. This happens because children are still primarily involved in their families of origin and therefore do not consistently displace these feelings to their treating physician or therapist. A flexible approach to the therapy, awareness of cultural differences in the child's background, and adjustments to meet the child's level of understanding are important features of successful treatment. **(p. 850)**

3. Which of the following is considered a working psychological explanation of the patient's feelings, behaviors, and thinking?

A. Assessment.
B. Diagnosis.
C. Formulation.
D. Conceptualization.

The correct response is Option C: Formulation.

In conducting a diagnostic evaluation of a child and initially interviewing parents and sometimes siblings, the clinician reaches two important conclusions: diagnosis and formulation. Each is equally meaningful in deciding how to help a young person with a mental disorder or developmental disturbance. The *formulation* consists of a working psychological explanation of the patient's feelings, behaviors, and thinking. *Assessment* is a process that leads to diagnosis and formulation. *Conceptualization* is a general term that describes understanding clinical material in the context of all of the information that is gathered. **(p. 851)**

4. Which of the following is most likely not very useful or effective in therapy when a child is not talking much in the early sessions?

A. Asking questions about the child's life.
B. Sitting quietly with the child so that they can feel empowered to talk.
C. Talking at length about video games the child might be playing at home.
D. Playing a game that does not require any talking.

The correct response is Option B: Sitting quietly with the child so that they can feel empowered to talk.

Most young people do not have much to say in the early stages of treatment, and it is often a good idea for the therapist to use conversation via an interactive game or talking about the child's life rather than waiting for the child to speak. Asking questions about the child's life, talking at length about video games the child might be playing at home, and playing a game that does not require the child to talk are some ways that might be helpful in engaging a child patient who is reluctant to converse. **(p. 856)**

5.   The role of parents in the child's individual psychotherapy can be varied but should always include which of the following?

A. Informing the parent(s) of what is troubling their child.
B. Discussing with the parent(s) the potential impact of significant events in the session.
C. The therapist being conscientious and thorough in deciding what to share with the parent(s).
D. The parent(s) having ongoing awareness of the goals and progress of the therapy.

The correct response is Option D: The parent(s) having ongoing awareness of the goals and progress of the therapy.

Parents need to understand, in an ongoing fashion, what the individual psychotherapy with their child is attempting to accomplish and where the accomplishment presently stands. The other options relate to breaches in confidentiality. **(p. 856)**

6.   The following are important and helpful considerations when terminating therapy with a child *except*

A. Taking into consideration whether the primary and secondary goals of treatment have been met.
B. Tapering the frequency of therapy sessions leading to termination.
C. Discussing termination when the family feels that the child has shown improvement.
D. Avoiding providing occasional booster sessions because this may be confusing to the child.

The correct response is Option D: Avoiding providing occasional booster sessions because this may be confusing to the child.

In fact, it is often useful for the clinician to make it clear that "booster shots" or subsequent briefer treatment periods may be necessary as the child goes through new developmental stages. All of the other options may be helpful in the process of termination. **(p. 868)**

CHAPTER 39

Parent Counseling, Psychoeducation, and Parent Support Groups

Jennifer B. Reese, Psy.D.

Mary A. Fristad, Ph.D., ABPP

1. The term *psychoeducation* refers to a wide range of interventions. Psychoeducation initially emerged to improve the prognosis of which disorder?

    A. Bipolar disorder.
    B. Anorexia nervosa.
    C. Selective mutism.
    D. Schizophrenia.

    The correct response is Option D: Schizophrenia.

    Goldstein et al. (1978) enrolled adults with schizophrenia who were recently discharged from a hospital and their family members in a program designed to help them understand the diagnosis, treatment, and crisis planning. The program was the first to combine medication and family intervention, which was found to be more effective than either alone. Psychoeducation as a technique can cover a wide range of topics such as diagnoses, course of illness, and medications and can serve as an adjunct to any other treatment. Although studies have been conducted to assess the use of psychoeducation in the treatment of bipolar disorder and eating disorders, including anorexia nervosa, these were developed later, after the initial use of psychoeducation for treatment of schizophrenia. There are no published studies on the use of psychoeducation for treatment of selective mutism. **(p. 875)**

2.   Which of the following terms refers to the type and quality of family members' interactions and attitudes regarding a person who has a mental illness?

A. Emotional energy.
B. Emotional intelligence.
C. Expressed emotion.
D. Ego explanation.

The correct response is Option C: Expressed emotion.

Psychoeducation can target *expressed emotion* (EE), which may contribute to the perpetuation of symptoms. EE refers to the type and quality of interactions and attitudes regarding a person who has a mental illness. This term emerged from a series of studies that found that high familial EE was associated with relapse rates in adults with schizophrenia (Brown et al. 1972). High EE has been identified as a risk factor for depression onset (Burkhouse et al. 2012) and has been found to relate to poor outcomes in youth with mood disorders (Asarnow et al. 1993).

Emotional energy is a term used by Levy (1939) to describe the importance of play because it reveals the inner world of the child and releases "emotional energy."

Emotional intelligence usually refers to one's perception and ability to handle emotions. There are other interventions targeting emotional intelligence.

The term *ego explanation* refers to how ego can be interpreted in the context of psychodynamic psychotherapy (such as coping or defenses) when a child has unwanted or "bad" behavior. **(p. 878)**

3.   Which of the following can be targets or topics of multifamily psychoeducational psychotherapy (MF-PEP) for both children and parents?

A. Medications, problem-solving skills, and mood disorders and family life.
B. Medications, systems of care, and communication.
C. Medications, symptom management techniques, and systems of care.
D. Medications, problem-solving skills, and communication.

The correct response is Option D: Medications, problem-solving skills, and communication.

MF-PEP consists of an 8-week curriculum designed for children (or adolescents) and caregivers. Each session begins with children and parents together, and then they are separated. Ideally, the child group is led by two co-therapists and the parent group by one therapist. At the end, parent and child groups rejoin for a wrap-up. The following topics are covered in both parent and child groups: medications, problem-solving skills, symptom management techniques, and communication. Systems of care and "mood disorders and family life" are topics for parent groups only. MF-PEP was initially developed as an adjunctive intervention for families with children ages 8–12 who have a mood disorder (Fristad et al. 2003). It was subsequently extended to adolescents and their parents and for a variety of conditions, including ADHD, autism spectrum disorder, disruptive behavior disorders, eating disorders, and trauma- and stressor-related disorders. **(p. 886; p. 887, Table 39–7)**

4. Compared with a wait list control group, youth in a study who received MF-PEP experienced which of the following?

    A. No change in mood symptoms.
    B. Worsening of mood symptoms.
    C. Decrease in mood symptom severity.
    D. Remission of mood symptoms.

    The correct response is Option C: Decrease in mood symptom severity.

    Fristad et al. (2009) found that youth who received MF-PEP had a significantly greater decrease in mood symptom severity at follow-up compared with a wait list control group. This improvement was maintained through an 18-month follow-up period. Studies suggest that MF-PEP helps parents become better consumers of mental health services by increasing their knowledge about mood disorders and treatment, which leads them to access higher-quality services. **(p. 886)**

5. All of the following reflect responsibilities of a support group facilitator *except*

    A. Allowing participants to share whatever is troubling them.
    B. Managing logistics.
    C. Creating a safe environment.
    D. Referring members to resources.

    The correct response is Option A: Allowing participants to share whatever is troubling them.

    Support group facilitators must moderate parental sharing during discussions, particularly to ensure that other group members are not overwhelmed. Not doing so can lead to several problems, including but not limited to group members sharing too much and inducing guilt in others that they "do not have it so bad" or members developing a "more unfortunate than thou" contest. There are additional risks without such moderation (e.g., members feel reluctant to share enough to allow an appropriate response, members share their success to the point of others feeling inferior). **(p. 890, Table 39–11; p. 893, Table 39–12)**

References

Asarnow JR, Goldstein MJ, Tompson M, et al: One-year outcomes of depressive disorders in child psychiatric in-patients: evaluation of the prognostic power of a brief measure of expressed emotion. J Child Psychol Psychiatry 34(2):129–137, 1993 8444988

Brown GW, Birley JL, Wing JK: Influence of family life on the course of schizophrenic disorders: a replication. Br J Psychiatry 121(562):241–258, 1972 5073778

Burkhouse KL, Uhrlass DJ, Stone LB, et al: Expressed emotion-criticism and risk of depression onset in children. J Clin Child Adolesc Psychol 41(6):771–777, 2012

Fristad MA, Gavazzi SM, Mackinaw-Koons B: Family psychoeducation: an adjunctive intervention for children with bipolar disorder. Biol Psychiatry 53(11):1000–1008, 2003 12788245

Fristad MA, Verducci JS, Walters K, et al: Impact of multifamily psychoeducational psychotherapy in treating children aged 8 to 12 years with mood disorders. Arch Gen Psychiatry 66(9):1013–1021, 2009 19736358

Goldstein MJ, Rodnick EH, Evans JR, et al: Drug and family therapy in the aftercare of acute schizophrenics. Arch Gen Psychiatry 35(10):1169–1177, 1978 211983

Levy D: Release therapy. Am J Orthopsychiatry 9:713–736, 1939

C H A P T E R   4 0

Behavioral Parent Training

Melissa R. Dvorsky, Ph.D.
Amanda Steinberg, B.S.

1. A parent engages in "special time" with their son by putting together a puzzle. The child attempts to fit an edge piece into the center. What should the parent do in response?

    A. Let the child figure out where the puzzle piece fits on his own.
    B. Ask the child questions about the puzzle piece to provide guidance.
    C. Hand the child another piece and explain why it fits better.
    D. Redirect the child to start with an easier section of the puzzle.

    The correct response is Option A: Let the child figure out where the piece fits on his own.

    Attending is meant to improve the parent-child relationship, and "special time" is used as an opportunity for the parent to actively attend to their child's behavior. Parents are encouraged to let the child direct the activity to the greatest extent possible in order for the child to feel that the activity is enjoyable and validating. Asking questions and praising and redirecting the child are all subtle ways of controlling the situation and consequently are to be avoided during the attending or special time exercise. **(pp. 907–908)**

2. Which of the following is *not* recommended for monitoring treatment progress in behavioral parent training?

    A. The clinician asks parents, "What rewards did your child earn and how often?"
    B. The clinician reviews the child's home behavior chart or daily report card data.
    C. The clinician observes parent-child interactions in a clean-up activity.
    D. The clinician rates their perception of parent engagement.

The correct response is Option D: The clinician rates their perception of parent engagement.

Although the provider's perception of a parent's engagement may be helpful information, that alone should not be used to inform treatment management because this perception can be subject to bias and the clinician may overlook key information. In behavior therapy, treatment progress is most effectively monitored by reviewing data (i.e., the child's progress on home behavior charts and daily report cards). Qualitative parent and teacher impressions on treatment progress provide objective idiographic data obtained by asking specific questions about how they are implementing the program and how the child is responding. Brief behavior ratings such as the Top Problems Assessment (Weisz et al. 2011) or questionnaires regarding parents' understanding of social learning principles and effective parenting practices can also be used to track progress. Asking parents specific questions to determine how well they are implementing the strategies provides a better assessment of treatment progress. **(pp. 919–920)**

3.   A mother is finishing dinner at home when her son, Dillon, begins to throw a tantrum. Exhausted from her day at work, the mother tries to get Dillon to quiet down quickly, saying she will give him a dessert if he calms down. Dillon stops and is provided dessert. What will this situation likely result in?

A. An increase in tantrums.
B. A decrease in tantrums.
C. A static trend in tantrums.
D. There is not enough information to determine the future trend of Dillon's tantrums.

The correct response is Option A: An increase in tantrums.

This case is an example of the misuse of rewards. Rewarding the termination of problem behavior may inadvertently increase that behavior through reinforcement. Therefore, the child's tantrums will likely increase if he knows that he will get dessert at some point after starting a tantrum. In this case, an appropriate use of a response cost procedure would be to be direct in taking away dessert privileges in the presence of a tantrum and rewarding dessert privileges in the absence of one. Alternatively, for more minor outbursts and mild negative behavior, the parent could use ignoring, as long as they are able to continue ignoring even if the behavior increases ("extinction burst"). If the parent gives in to the child before the negative behavior stops, that behavior will likely increase in the future. **(pp. 915, 920)**

4.   Mrs. Adams is on her third week of using a token economy reward system with her son, Ben. Ben struggles with getting his homework done after school, so his goal is to complete his homework before 4:00 P.M. with no more than one reminder. Ben fulfilled his homework routine after school in the first week to earn all points on his behavioral reward chart. However, in the second and third weeks, Mrs. Adams had to give multiple reminders, and he earned his daily reward only

once. Ben and his mother are frustrated, and Ben repeatedly complains that the behavioral reward chart is not going to work. What would be the most appropriate next step for Mrs. Adams to address this?

A. Stop implementing the token economy and consider other behavioral parenting strategies.
B. Restate to Ben what his goals are and see how he responds.
C. Increase the criterion from one reminder for completing his homework to two or three reminders.
D. Do nothing and allow more time for Ben to adjust to the new system.

The correct response is Option C: Increase the criterion from one reminder for completing his homework to two or three reminders.

When the assessment of progress shows that desired effects of the structured rewards system are not achieved, it is important to assess how well parents are implementing the program and how well the child responds to the program. Sometimes, the treatment criteria are set too high, and the child may display more success if the criteria for their performance are more realistic. Goals can gradually increase in difficulty as youth show consistent success with their set criteria. In the case of Mrs. Adams, the behavioral goal criterion of no more than one reminder for his homework may be unrealistic for Ben to start with, and increasing the number of reminders to two or three may set Ben up for success.

Other forms of treatment can be appropriate to address problems within the family system (e.g., marital therapy, treatment for parental ADHD). These adjunctive treatments can occur concurrently with behavioral parent training, or parent training can be paused temporarily until gains in alternative treatments are achieved. If, at first, the only presenting problem is that the goals set are too difficult to reach, then setting more realistic goals would be the appropriate initial plan of action.

Although parents need to reiterate their child's goals throughout implementing behavior treatment and leave room for adjustment, this program is meant to be feasible and holds many opportunities for quick success and immediate rewards. **(pp. 921–922)**

5. Which of the following factors is least likely to influence behavioral intervention treatment outcomes?

A. Parents with low socioeconomic status.
B. The number of children in a family.
C. Single-parent families.
D. Parents who believe that their child is behaving badly on purpose.

The correct response is Option B: The number of children in a family.

The number of children at home is not necessarily associated with outcomes of behavioral parent training. There is more robust empirical support for the effect of the other family factors noted.

Generally, the more difficult the home living conditions and the more impaired the relationship between the child and parent, the less favorable the outcome. Past research suggests that low socioeconomic status (SES) is a significant barrier to effective care. Low levels of SES can lead to limited access and support for families, and those stressors experienced by low-SES families contribute to a greater likelihood of early termination from behavioral parent training.

Single-parent families and families with high parent stress predict less favorable outcomes. In addition, if parents believe that their child is trying to behave poorly on purpose or is destined to display negative behavior, they are often less likely to feel motivated to implement new behavioral strategies. Having multiple children can lead to greater caregiver strain, and it is important to discuss how behavioral strategies will be implemented in a home with other children, especially when they are close in age. **(pp. 925–926)**

6. The triad of disorders identified as disruptive behavior disorders that behavioral parent training was developed to address most commonly includes the following DSM-5 (American Psychiatric Association 2013) diagnoses *except* which of the following?

A. ADHD.
B. Oppositional defiant disorder.
C. Obsessive-compulsive disorder.
D. Conduct disorder.

The correct response is Option C: Obsessive-compulsive disorder

Although DSM-5 no longer classifies ADHD as a disruptive behavior disorder (it is grouped under the neurodevelopmental disorders category), in the development of behavioral parent training, the triad of disorders consisting of ADHD, oppositional defiant disorder, and conduct disorder are referred to as disruptive behavior disorders. These specific disorders display a lack of sensitivity to partial reinforcement, elevated reward thresholds, a marked aversion to delays in reinforcement, and reduced responsiveness to cues of punishment or nonreward. **(p. 901)**

References

American Psychiatric Association: Diagnostic and Statistical Manual of Mental Disorders, 5th Edition. Arlington, VA, American Psychiatric Association, 2013
Weisz JR, Chorpita BF, Frye A, et al: Youth top problems: using idiographic, consumer-guided assessment to identify treatment needs and track change during psychotherapy. J Consult Clin Psychol 79(3):369–380, 2011 21500888

CHAPTER 41

Family-Based Assessment and Treatment

Karen R. Gouze, Ph.D.

Richard Wendel, Ph.D.

1.   A 5-year-old boy, accompanied by his parents, presents in your office with several symptoms, including temper tantrums, high levels of negative affect, and reluctance to attend school. All of the following would be the benefits of family therapy *except*

A. Improved parenting skills.
B. Reduction in symptoms.
C. Parent satisfaction with the treatment.
D. Improvement in symptoms of ADHD.

The correct response is Option D: Improvement in symptoms of ADHD.

A child with moderate to severe ADHD might require pharmacological intervention before significant progress can be made through family therapy. In a meta-analysis of published studies involving family support in children's mental health (Hoagwood et al. 2010), it was found that when parent support was integrated into child treatment, overall results were positive for child symptom reduction, parental satisfaction with the treatment, improved parenting skills, parental knowledge of the child's illness, and perceived social support. **(pp. 933–934, 941)**

2. Which of the following options is a more important focus in family therapy than in individual therapy?

A. The child's symptoms.
B. The parent's symptoms.
C. Patterns of interaction that create or contribute to the child's symptoms.
D. Normal developmental processes.

The correct response is Option C: Patterns of interaction that create or contribute to the child's symptoms.

Although the child's symptoms and the parent's symptoms could be part of the family therapy process, these are not the main focus. Patterns of interaction that create or contribute to the child's symptoms are more important in family therapy than in individual therapy. Although normal developmental processes should be considered by a clinician, they are not the major focus in family therapy. **(p. 935)**

3. Which of the following is an important family variable that contributes to externalizing behavior in children?

A. Clear parental boundaries.
B. Parental hostility.
C. Sibling rivalry.
D. Living with extended family members.

The correct response is Option B: Parental hostility.

The formative role played by families in promoting or attenuating mental health in children has been well documented in the developmental psychopathology literature. For example, in both preschoolers and school-age children, a strong relationship is found between externalizing behaviors and family variables, including conflict, parental psychopathology, parental hostility and warmth, and parental scaffolding (Grant et al. 2006; Lavigne et al. 2016). Although parental boundaries, sibling rivalry, and the presence of extended family members are important aspects of one's family and may contribute to behavioral disturbance, there is no evidence to suggest a clear correlation between these factors and externalizing behavior. **(p. 937)**

4. A family comes to your office for the treatment of their 14-year-old son. When you ask what brings them to therapy, they launch into a long list of grievances about their child, including his substance use, disrespect, failing grades, and use of unacceptable language. In family therapy, this presentation is considered to be which of the following?

A. A problem-saturated narrative.
B. A family-based description of the problem.

C. A contextually sensitive narrative.

D. A well-formulated problem description.

The correct response is Option A: A problem-saturated narrative.

Successful family-based treatments share specific characteristics. In therapies for individuals, when the patient enters the consultation room, it is reasonable for the clinician to ask, in a variety of ways, "What is the problem?" Working with dyads and families requires different tactics. Families, by definition, involve multiple people, often with different experiences and perspectives on the problem. Clinicians who ask a family "What is the problem?" are likely to hear the most verbal and most frustrated person, probably a parent, launch into a problem-saturated description, such as that portrayed in this case example. The other options do not describe this scenario. **(p. 939)**

5.   Which of the following is *not* part of the family therapy technique known as *joining*?

A. Avoid the "What's wrong?" question.

B. Start with relationship-building small talk with each person in the room.

C. Avoid talking about serious problems until everyone has a chance to connect with the therapist.

D. Immediately discuss the serious issues as soon as they are talked about, even if everyone in attendance has not had a chance to enter the process.

The correct response is Option D: Immediately discuss the serious issues as soon as they are talked about, even if everyone in attendance has not had a chance to enter the process.

Family therapists actively use a technique known as *joining*. There are three principles of joining: 1) avoid the "What's wrong?" question, 2) begin with relationship-building small talk with each person in the room, and 3) postpone discussion of the serious issues until everyone in attendance has had a chance to enter the process. Following this joining with the family, the therapist solicits each person's view of the problem in turn. It is wise to move on to the next stage only after everyone's story has been heard. **(p. 940)**

6.   Integrative Module-Based Family Therapy (IMBFT) is best described as which of the following?

A. An integrative approach to family therapy.

B. A psychoanalytic approach to family therapy.

C. A cognitive-behavioral approach to family therapy.

D. A psychiatric/biological approach to family therapy.

The correct response is Option A: An integrative approach to family therapy.

The IMBFT approach combines previous integrative family therapy models with empirically supported and best practice approaches to family treatment and theoretical and empirical knowledge from the fields of developmental psychology and psychopathology, family studies, and psychiatry to provide a road map for assessment and treatment of families (Gouze and Wendel 2008; Wendel and Gouze 2010). IMBFT is not a psychoanalytic, cognitive-behavioral, or biological approach to family therapy. **(p. 941)**

7.   *Reframing* is a technique used in which of the following domains of IMBFT?

A. The attachment/relationship domain.
B. The mastery domain.
C. The cognitive/narrative domain.
D. The affect regulation domain.

The correct response is Option C: The cognitive/narrative domain.

IMBFT describes 10 areas referred to as domains in which there are empirically established or reasonably assumed mechanisms of change. These 10 domains are the psychiatric/biological domain, attachment/relationship domain, family structure domain, family communication domain, developmental domain, affect regulation domain, behavior regulation domain, cognitive/narrative domain, mastery domain, and community domain.

The cognitive/narrative domain is addressed first if family stories or myths continue to support maladaptive behavior in an individual child or adolescent (e.g., "He's the lazy one in the family"). Or it might be the first domain engaged in intervention if cognitive restructuring is required to shift a family's focus from a problem-focused view of a child to the things they do right. Reframing, a time-honored technique in family therapy in which a more positive perspective is placed on what is otherwise seen as a maladaptive behavior, falls in this category. An example might be when a mother complains that an anxious child is "driving me crazy" with her clingy behavior, and the therapist reframes this as the child's need to be close to her mother. **(pp. 941–943)**

References

Gouze KR, Wendel R: Integrative module-based family therapy: application and training. J Marital Fam Ther 34(3):269–286, 2008 18717919

Grant KE, Compas BE, Thurm AE, et al: Stressors and child and adolescent psychopathology: evidence of moderating and mediating effects. Clin Psychol Rev 26(3):257–283, 2006 16364522

Hoagwood KE, Cavaleri MA, Olin SS, et al: Family support in children's mental health: a review and synthesis. Clin Child Fam Psychol Rev 13(1):1–45, 2010 20012893

Lavigne JV, Gouze KR, Hopkins J, Bryant FB: A multidomain cascade model of early childhood risk factors associated with oppositional defiant disorder symptoms in a community sample of 6-year-olds. Dev Psychopathol 28 (4 pt 2):1547–1562, 2016

Wendel R, Gouze KR: Family therapy: assessment and intervention, in Dulcan's Textbook of Child and Adolescent Psychiatry. Edited by Dulcan MK. Washington, DC, American Psychiatric Publishing, 2010, pp 869–886

CHAPTER 42

Interpersonal Psychotherapy for Depressed Adolescents

Meredith L. Gunlicks-Stoessel, Ph.D.
Laura Mufson, Ph.D.

1. The therapist explains to an adolescent with depression and her parents that it is important for the teen to do as many of her activities as possible, such as getting to school, doing homework, and participating in after-school activities, but with the awareness and acceptance that the teen might not do these things as often or as well as before the depression developed. What is this explanation called?

    A. Behavioral activation.
    B. Cognitive restructuring.
    C. Increasing pleasurable activities.
    D. Limited sick role.

    The correct response is Option D: Limited sick role.

    The limited sick role aims to balance encouraging engagement in as many usual or expected activities as possible with an awareness and acceptance that performance will likely be reduced. The aim is to reduce expectations and then to be able to increase them as the depressive symptoms remit. In addition, in sharing the concept of the limited sick role with the parent, the goal is to help the parent to take a more encouraging and supportive stance rather than a critical one toward the adolescent's current level of performance. Behavioral activation focuses on increasing engagement in pleasurable activities to improve mood, whereas cognitive restructuring focuses on noticing and changing unhelpful thinking patterns. **(p. 957)**

2.   Which of the following describes the closeness circle in interpersonal psychotherapy?

   A. It is helpful in the middle phase to assist in role-play.
   B. It is used to identify relationships and guide the interpersonal inventory.
   C. It illustrates how the adolescent's depression symptoms affect their relationships.
   D. It is completed as part of homework in the initial phase of treatment.

   The correct response is Option B: It is used to identify relationships and guide the interpersonal inventory.

   The closeness circle is a series of four concentric circles; the therapist writes the adolescent's name in the center, then writes the names of the people in the adolescent's life, placed according to the closeness of their relationship. The closeness circle is used to identify the important people in the adolescent's life about whom the therapist will ask questions during the interpersonal inventory. The therapist and adolescent complete the closeness circle together during a session in the initial phase of treatment. Identifying the link between mood and relationships is not a part of the closeness circle; rather, the therapist and adolescent will discuss how the adolescent's symptoms of depression affect their relationships during the interpersonal inventory. Names are written in each concentric circle on the basis of how close the relationship is rather than how much the relationship is related to the adolescent's mood. **(p. 957)**

3.   A teenage girl became depressed after her mother's remarriage, their subsequent move to a new community, and the inclusion of stepsisters in the home. She and her mother have not been getting along well since the move. Which of the following is the best description of her struggles according to the interpersonal psychotherapy model?

   A. Grief.
   B. Interpersonal deficits.
   C. Interpersonal role disputes.
   D. Interpersonal role transitions.

   The correct response is Option D: Interpersonal role transitions.

   This teenager has experienced a life change that requires her to alter her behavior from an old role to a new role (living in a new household with a new stepparent and stepsiblings and living in a new community). The onset of her symptoms of depression coincides with this life change, and thus the problem area of interpersonal role transitions is assigned. Her depressive symptoms are not associated with the death of a loved one or due to globally underdeveloped social and communication skills that impair her ability to have positive relationships. Although the teenager has not been getting along well with her mother, this developed after the move and would be considered part of the role transition rather than an independent problem area of interpersonal role disputes. **(p. 958)**

4.   Which of the following is *not* a goal for the problem area of interpersonal role disputes?

A. Gain interpersonal problem-solving skills to resolve the dispute.
B. Identify the teen's expectations for the other person and the other person's expectations for the teen.
C. Mourn the loss of how the relationship used to be.
D. Gain communication skills to resolve the dispute.

The correct response is Option C: Mourn the loss of how the relationship used to be.

The goal of working in the problem area of role disputes is to try to find a path to resolution of the disagreement or nonreciprocal expectations for the relationship. To do that, strategies include clarifying expectations for the relationship and improving the adolescent's skills in communication and problem-solving, as needed. Mourning the loss of the relationship and how it was experienced in the past is a strategy more aligned with working with role transitions in which something has changed and the adolescent is having difficulty accepting the change and the new role that has resulted from the transition. **(pp. 958, 961)**

5.   All of the following techniques are used in interpersonal psychotherapy for depressed adolescents (IPT-A) *except*

A. Communication analysis.
B. Cognitive restructuring.
C. Role-playing.
D. Decision analysis.

The correct response is Option B: Cognitive restructuring.

Cognitive restructuring is a therapeutic technique that is used in cognitive-behavioral therapy. It focuses on reframing negative thoughts about a situation into a more positive outlook. In contrast, in IPT-A, the focus is not initially on changing negative thoughts but rather on changing the interpersonal interaction by altering communication strategies or the approach to problem-solving. Therefore, communication analysis is an important technique for dissecting interactions into verbal and nonverbal communications to understand what changes might be needed. Decision analysis is IPT-A's approach to problem-solving, and role-playing in IPT-A helps patients practice new interpersonal skills within the safety of the session before using them in situations outside the therapy room. **(p. 960)**

6.   Which of the following is not one of the tasks for the termination phase of treatment with interpersonal psychotherapy?

A. Share feelings about ending the relationship with the therapist.
B. Review strategies that were practiced during treatment.

C. Review warning signs of depression.

D. Review mood ratings and events that could affect mood ratings in the future.

The correct response is Option D: Review mood ratings and events that could affect mood ratings in the future.

The tasks for the termination phase are 1) help the adolescent to express feelings about the end of treatment, including positive and negative feelings about treatment and any concerns about ending the treatment, 2) review the specific treatment strategies used in IPT-A, 3) discuss the experiences in using the strategies and how they might be helpful in future situations, 4) identify signs that the adolescent might experience a recurrence of depression, and 5) assess the need for further treatment. Reviewing mood ratings and associated events is not a primary task of the termination phase of treatment. The adolescent's personal symptom profile is reviewed to identify the salient symptoms that should alert the teen to reach out for help in the future. **(p. 962)**

CHAPTER 43

Cognitive-Behavioral Treatment for Anxiety and Depression

Ashley Winch, M.S.

1. Why is parental involvement in cognitive-behavioral therapy (CBT) an integral part of treatment?

    A. Parental involvement in treatment aids in the development of appropriate goals for treatment.
    B. Parental involvement in treatment aids in the teaching and implementation of the skills learned in treatment.
    C. Parental involvement in treatment can lead to more effective parenting practices that can increase the likelihood of remission.
    D. All of the above.

    The correct response is Option D: All of the above.

    Parental involvement in CBT is integral to the success of treatment for anxiety and depression in children and adolescents. Including parents in the treatment process helps in the development of treatment goals, aids in teaching and implementation of skills learned in treatment, and encourages more effective parenting practices. **(pp. 976–979)**

2. A 12-year-old patient begins treatment for injection phobia. You determine that CBT is the optimal treatment method for this youth. Because of his fear of being given an injection, the patient has such intense anxiety that he refuses to leave the

house if he is aware that there will be a doctor's appointment. What would be a potentially appropriate early step in a graduated exposure for this patient?

A. Relaxation training.
B. Showing him a picture of someone like him receiving an injection.
C. Teaching him how to engage in cognitive restructuring.
D. Driving him to the doctor's office without telling him where he is going.

The correct response is Option B: Showing him a picture of someone like him receiving an injection.

Relaxation training and cognitive restructuring are important components of CBT for children and adolescents with anxiety or depression. However, relaxation training is discouraged when engaging in graduated exposure because the youth needs to tolerate the distress and learn that it will dissipate.

Showing the patient a picture of someone like him receiving an injection is an appropriate early step in graduated exposure because seeing the picture is potentially distressing enough that the patient experiences anxiety but distant enough that the anxiety is not overwhelming. In this way, the patient can practice distress tolerance and build his confidence to try a more anxiety-inducing step on the hierarchy.

Driving the patient to the doctor's office without his knowledge is not an appropriate step in the hierarchy. The patient, parent(s), and therapist should work collaboratively to develop the graduated exposure hierarchy. Part of the rationale is that each step of the hierarchy is anxiety inducing, but the patient will resist the urge to avoid the situation and will learn distress tolerance. Exposing the patient to the doctor's office without his knowledge would be inappropriate and potentially overwhelming. **(pp. 968–969)**

3. Social skills training may be an important component of CBT for children and adolescents in treatment for which of the following?

A. Depression but not social anxiety.
B. Generalized anxiety without social anxiety.
C. Social anxiety but not depression.
D. Depression or social anxiety.

The correct response is Option D: Depression or social anxiety.

Social skills training may be an important component of CBT for children and adolescents in treatment for depression and/or social anxiety, whether separately or comorbid. It is important to remember that components of treatment can be beneficial for multiple diagnoses. Social skills training will also help treat patients with comorbid generalized anxiety and social anxiety. **(pp. 970–972)**

4. With regard to mood monitoring as an intervention for a child or an adolescent with depression, which of the following is beneficial for them to monitor?

A. Any of their negative moods.
B. Their negative and positive moods.
C. Their depression-related moods.
D. Their depression- or anxiety-related moods.

The correct response is Option B: Their negative and positive moods.

It is important for children and adolescents experiencing depression to monitor their negative moods; however, it is beneficial for them to also monitor their positive moods. By monitoring positive moods in addition to negative moods, the youth will better understand the lability of their moods and how they change in response to events. **(p. 970)**

5. The Child/Adolescent Anxiety Multimodal Study (CAMS; Walkup et al. 2008) was a randomized controlled trial that examined the efficacy of CBT, pharmacological intervention, a combination of CBT and pharmacological intervention, and pill placebo for children and adolescents with anxiety. The Treatment for Adolescents With Depression Study (TADS; March et al. 2004; Treatment for Adolescents With Depression Study Team 2003) used the same model to determine the efficacy of these treatments in adolescents with depression. Which of the following accurately describes the findings from these studies?

A. The combination of CBT and pharmacological intervention resulted in the highest remission rates.
B. Pharmacological intervention resulted in the highest remission rates.
C. The combination of CBT and pharmacological intervention resulted in the highest initial remission rates.
D. CBT intervention resulted in the highest remission rates.

The correct response is Option C: The combination of CBT and pharmacological intervention resulted in the highest initial remission rates.

It is important to remember that although CBT and pharmacological interventions have been demonstrated to be efficacious treatments for youth with depression or anxiety, a large portion of youth do not respond to either treatment or to both treatments combined. The consistent finding across the studies was that the combination of CBT and pharmacological intervention resulted in the highest initial remission rates. When pharmacological treatment and CBT interventions were given separately, remission rates were lower than in the group assigned to combined treatment. Interestingly, when the youth in these studies were followed longitudinally, the initial treatment condition was not predictive of remission over time. **(pp. 971–974)**

References

March J, Silva S, Petrycki S, et al: Fluoxetine, cognitive-behavioral therapy, and their combination for adolescents with depression: Treatment for Adolescents With Depression Study (TADS) randomized controlled trial. JAMA 292(7):807–820, 2004 15315995

Treatment for Adolescents With Depression Study Team: Treatment for Adolescents With Depression Study (TADS): rationale, design, and methods. J Am Acad Child Adolesc Psychiatry 42(5):531–542, 2003 12707557

Walkup JT, Albano AM, Piacentini J, et al: Cognitive behavioral therapy, sertraline, or a combination in childhood anxiety. N Engl J Med 359(26):2753–2766, 2008 18974308

CHAPTER 44

Motivational Interviewing

Kelly Walker Lowry, Ph.D.

1. All of the following are true regarding motivational interviewing (MI) *except*

    A. According to a meta-analysis, 75% of participants benefit from MI.
    B. MI has a proven role in treating youth substance use and youth with psychiatric comorbidities.
    C. MI has known utility in pediatric behavioral health concerns, including in patients with diabetes or asthma.
    D. MI studies have found larger effect sizes with ethnic majority youth compared with minority youth.

    The correct response is Option D: MI studies have found larger effect sizes with ethnic majority youth compared with minority youth.

    The effectiveness of MI across a wide variety of targets is well established. A meta-analysis representing 119 studies concluded that 75% of participants benefited from MI, with 50% obtaining a small but meaningful effect and 25% obtaining a moderate or strong effect from MI interventions (Lundahl et al. 2010). Evidence in child and adolescent psychiatry includes support for MI in the treatment of youth substance use (Naar-King 2011), youth with psychiatric comorbidities (Brown et al. 2015), and pediatric behavioral health concerns, including patients with diabetes or asthma (Gayes and Steele 2014), as well as in schools (Rollnick et al. 2016) and juvenile justice settings (Stein 2010). Although results of subgroup research on MI are mixed, studies have found larger effect sizes with minority youth compared with ethnic majority youth (Hettema et al. 2005). **(pp. 985–986)**

2. According to the MI model, which of the following terms describes the concept that the therapist and client are equal experts?

A. Acceptance.
B. Compassion.
C. Partnership.
D. Evocation.

The correct response is Option C: Partnership.

In MI, partnership is a concept proposing that both the therapist and the client are equal experts. The therapist is an expert guide in helping people change, and clients are experts on their reasons for change, their ideas about how to change, their communities, and themselves.

Acceptance refers to a conscious decision on the therapist's part to recognize client autonomy in making decisions. Acceptance is differentiated in this model from tacit approval, and clinicians may at times speak of that distinction directly.

Compassion is the active process of promoting and holding the client's welfare as paramount and prioritizing the client's best interests and needs.

Evocation is the process by which factors internal to the client are called forth and elicited. In MI, evocation is an active process, starting from a strengths-focused assumption that people have within them what they need and that the therapist's role is to evoke it rather than providing it. **(p. 986)**

3. Which of the following options correctly describes OARS, the four MI processes?

A. Optimism, adaptations, reflections, and summaries.
B. Open-ended questions, affirmations, reflections, and summaries.
C. Object relations, affirmations, reflections, and summaries.
D. Open-ended questions, adaptations, responsiveness, and summaries.

The correct response is Option B: Open-ended questions, affirmations, reflections, and summaries.

Clinicians familiar with MI use the following specific MI communication skills: open-ended questions, affirmations, reflections, and summaries (OARS). Although these approaches are not specific to MI, the strategic ways in which the OARS skills are applied are distinct to MI. **(pp. 986–988)**

4. Which of the following is true regarding MI?

A. MI is an example of an unstructured psychotherapy approach.
B. It is best not to combine MI with other approaches such as cognitive-behavioral therapy (CBT).
C. MI can be learned and competently practiced by clinicians from various disciplines.
D. MI requires highly specialized training that is not available to some disciplines.

The correct response is Option C: MI can be learned and competently practiced by clinicians from various disciplines.

MI is a structured, teachable, and effective process for helping people change. MI can be used in isolation or combined with other active or skills-based approaches, such as CBT. The blending of approaches may actually improve the effectiveness of each. Learning MI takes time, practice, and feedback, but it can be learned and competently practiced by clinicians from various disciplines. **(p. 997)**

5.   Which of the following is true regarding MI and group treatment?

A. MI should not be used as a group treatment at any age.
B. MI is effective in group treatment settings, including youth group treatment.
C. MI can be used as a group treatment with no distinction from other approaches for group treatment.
D. It is crucial for group members to demonstrate readiness for change for effective MI delivery.

The correct response is Option B: MI is effective in group treatment settings, including youth group treatment.

MI is effective in group treatment settings, including youth group treatment. Several factors distinguish MI groups from other types of group treatment. The first distinction is that the goal of an MI group is to guide a discussion that will lead to behavior change rather than simply to pass along knowledge. A second distinction is a focus on creating a space where youth can examine their motivations and ideas with autonomy.

MI can be useful as a group treatment regardless of the stage of readiness of group members. If group members express readiness, group leaders may explore planning for change with group members. However, this can be discussed in hypothetical scenarios if individual members are not yet ready for change. The evocation of plans and SMART goals (specific, measurable, achievable, realistic, timely) can be implemented for group members who are ready to take steps toward a specific change. **(pp. 991–992)**

References

Brown RA, Abrantes AM, Minami H, et al: Motivational interviewing to reduce substance use in adolescents with psychiatric comorbidity. J Subst Abuse Treat 59:20–29, 2015 26362000
Gayes LA, Steele RG: A meta-analysis of motivational interviewing interventions for pediatric health behavior change. J Consult Clin Psychol 82(3):521–535, 2014 24547922
Hettema J, Steele J, Miller WR: Motivational interviewing. Annu Rev Clin Psychol 1:91–111, 2005 17716083
Lundahl BW, Kunz C, Brownell C, et al: A meta-analysis of motivational interviewing: twenty-five years of empirical studies. Res Soc Work Pract 20(2):137–160, 2010

Naar-King S: Motivational interviewing in adolescent treatment. Can J Psychiatry 56(11):651–657, 2011 22114919

Rollnick S, Kaplan SG, Rutschman R: Motivational Interviewing in Schools: Conversations to Improve Behavior and Learning. New York, Guilford, 2016

Stein LAR: The juvenile justice system, in Motivational Interviewing With Adolescents and Young Adults. Edited by Naar-King S, Suarez M. New York, Guilford, 2010, pp 100–105

CHAPTER 45

Systems of Care, Wraparound Services, and Home-Based Services

Yann B. Poncin, M.D.

1. Which of the following best describes wraparound services?

    A. Wraparound services are a process for engaging with families to bring together an array of informal and formal community services to support the needs of a child and family.

    B. Wraparound services are a primary tool for engaging with families in Multisystemic Therapy (MST).

    C. Wraparound services are one of the four domains of clinical care used by Intensive In-Home Child and Adolescent Psychiatric Services (IICAPS).

    D. Wraparound services describes intakes conducted in which caregivers and other adults involved in a child's life are interviewed.

    The correct response is Option A: Wraparound services are a process for engaging with families to bring together an array of informal and formal community services to support the needs of a child and family.

    Wraparound services are a process for engaging with families using strength-based and culturally competent approaches that focus on bringing together both natural and formal supports, "wrapping" services in the community around a child and family according to their individual needs. MST and IICAPS are community- and home-based clinical treatment services that do not have a defined wraparound approach but may have elements that overlap with a wraparound philosophy. Intakes can include the interview of several informants, but that is not an example of a wraparound level of care. **(pp. 999, 1009–1010)**

2.   What is the system of care (SOC)?

A. The SOC refers to the school, child protection, judicial, and mental health treatment services within a given community.
B. The SOC comprises the informal and formal supports available in a given community, including as an integral part the linkage of supports and coordinating access to care.
C. The SOC describes the federal, state, county, and local mental health service system and its coordination.
D. The SOC represents the formal and informal support services that are coordinated across tribal organizations in the United States.

The correct response is Option B: The SOC comprises the informal and formal supports available in a given community, including as an integral part the linkage of supports and coordinating access to care.

Option A represents elements that might be part of a larger system of care because mental health services are often distributed across entities. The other options do not describe processes defined by the SOC. **(p. 999)**

3.   Each of the following options is a key feature of home-based or intensive home-based services *except*

A. 24-hour availability (24/7).
B. Services delivered in the community.
C. Psychiatric care.
D. Small caseloads.

The correct response is Option C: Psychiatric care.

Although the integration of or access to psychiatric care varies across types of services, psychiatric care is not considered a core component of home-based services. Home-based services are often an integral part of a system of care. Because of the resources, staffing, funding, and intensity of treatment that are required, home-based services are typically reserved for families who have children at risk of being placed out of home, whether in a hospital, residential treatment center, correctional facility, foster home, or other location. **(p. 1008)**

4.   Which of the following acts or programs is not related to the emerging provision of mental health care for children?

A. Mental Retardation Facilities and Community Mental Health Centers Construction Act.
B. Child and Adolescent Service System Program.

C. Comprehensive Community Mental Health Services for Children and Their Families Program.

D. Individuals with Disabilities Education Act.

The correct response is Option A: Mental Retardation Facilities and Community Mental Health Centers Construction Act.

The Mental Retardation Facilities and Community Mental Health Centers Construction Act of 1963 created a national network of community mental health centers. The act did not specifically address children, and only half of the centers had children's services. The other options describe acts or programs with varying direct positive efforts toward or affecting children. A goal of the Child and Adolescent Service System Program was to enable children with special needs to access services without resorting to the juvenile justice or child protective service systems for care. The Comprehensive Community Mental Health Services for Children and Their Families Program was created to promote the coordination of the multiple systems that serve children and youth from birth to age 21 years who are diagnosed with a serious emotional disturbance. The Individuals with Disabilities Education Act, originally known as the Education for All Handicapped Children Act of 1975, now defines 14 categories of educational disabilities. **(p. 1000)**

5. What was the intent of the Adoption Assistance and Child Welfare Act of 1980?

A. To provide better funding for foster care agencies.

B. To ameliorate the conditions in which children live before placement.

C. To provide better funding for foster care parents.

D. To strengthen permanency planning for children.

The correct response is Option D: To strengthen permanency planning for children.

The intent of the Adoption Assistance and Child Welfare Act of 1980 (P.L. 96-272) was to strengthen permanency planning for children. States are required to make efforts to prevent the removal of youth from their family or to return them to their family. If attempts to have a child remain with the family are unsuccessful, there must be permanency planning. In 1993, Congress passed legislation establishing Title IV, Part B-2 of the Social Security Act, creating funding for family preservation and family support programs. Although the other options are examples of concerns over the years, they do not apply to the Adoption Assistance and Child Welfare Act. **(p. 1008)**

CHAPTER 46

Milieu Treatment

Inpatient, Partial Hospitalization, and Residential Programs

Khushbu Shah, M.D., M.P.H.

1. What is the best way to prevent elopement and risky behaviors in milieu treatment programs?

    A. Effective communication.
    B. Smaller unit census.
    C. Active parental involvement in treatment.
    D. Availability of PRN medications.

    The correct response is Option A: Effective communication.

    Dynamics related to elopement from treatment programs are similar to those found in youth who exhibit self-injurious behavior (e.g., self-cutting, head banging, ingesting foreign objects). Effective communication among staff and between staff and patients is the best way to prevent elopement and other risky behaviors. The unit size is not known to be associated with elopement risk. Although parental involvement in treatment and as-needed medication availability are important aspects of treatment, they do not prevent elopement and risky behaviors. **(p. 1024)**

2. Readmission rate is one of the quality measures for inpatient units according to the Centers for Medicare and Medicaid Services and the Affordable Care Act. Return to hospitalization in which one of the following time frames defines readmission?

    A. 24 hours.
    B. 48 hours.

C. 30 days.
D. 60 days.

The correct response is Option C: 30 days.

Readmission rates have garnered increased attention because of the cost and other implications of inadequate outcomes of a hospitalization. The Centers for Medicare and Medicaid Services and the Affordable Care Act specify inpatient unit readmission in less than 30 days as a quality measure. **(p. 1025)**

3.   Which of the following factors is associated with a lower rehospitalization rate?

A. Longer inpatient hospitalization stays.
B. Longer period of day treatment.
C. Younger age of the patient.
D. Use of psychotropic medications.

The correct response is Option B: Longer period of day treatment.

Readmission rates to intensive services within 30 days of discharge are high. Risk factors include suicidal thoughts and behaviors, younger age, permissive or harsh parenting, caregiver-child conflict, long initial hospital stay, psychosis and suicide attempts, nonsuicidal self-injury in the month before admission for depressed youth, history of abuse and neglect or other trauma, and being in an adoptive home.

Solutions to readmission risk are being developed. According to a report by Trask et al. (2016), a lower rehospitalization rate was significantly related to both total service hours received postdischarge and receiving more days of day treatment. Although psychotropic medications are prescribed as indicated, the use of medications is not known to be associated with the rehospitalization rate. **(pp. 1025–1026)**

4.   Carter, a 14-year-old adolescent, presents with a history of depression and anxiety, with worsening symptoms in the context of several psychosocial stressors at home and school. His home environment is currently unstable, and his aunt, his primary caregiver, has recently needed to take on a second job because of financial stressors. Carter's aunt has not been able to provide consistent supervision for medication monitoring or take him to therapy appointments. In the past, Carter has decompensated when he was nonadherent to treatment recommendations or did not have close structure and supervision. He currently denies active suicidal ideation or self-injurious behaviors but has recently had some thoughts and urges. Which of the following is the most appropriate placement?

A. Acute inpatient psychiatric unit.
B. Partial hospitalization program.
C. Therapeutic day school.
D. Residential treatment center.

The correct response is Option D: Residential treatment center.

Children in residential treatment centers (RTCs) typically have been unable to be treated successfully as outpatients and frequently have needs related to food, shelter, school placement, and mental health and other health care. Presenting problems often include various combinations of family conflict or dysfunction, aggression, inability to succeed in school, depression, anxiety disorders, and delinquent behavior.

In residential treatment, more independent functioning is expected compared with hospital treatment, where total care is provided. In addition, RTCs expect "healthy" behavior compared with the "sick role" behavior allowed and expected during an acute inpatient hospital stay.

For successful partial hospital or day treatment care such as a therapeutic day school, parents or caregivers must be able to regularly participate in family counseling, training, and therapy and adequately provide support for and control over their children during evenings and weekends. Reliable transportation must also be available. **(pp. 1022, 1027, 1028, 1033)**

5. Which of the following is one of the two most common types of therapeutic modalities applied in therapeutic milieus?

    A. Dialectical behavioral therapy (DBT).
    B. Motivational interviewing (MI).
    C. Interpersonal psychotherapy (IPT).
    D. Parent management training (PMT).

The correct response is Option A: Dialectical behavioral therapy (DBT).

DBT techniques are increasingly used in many milieu treatment programs. These strategies are especially useful for suicidal and self-injurious youth by targeting impulsive aggression, noncompliance, and engagement in therapy.

DBT has been demonstrated to be feasible across clinical settings and a range of psychiatric disorders and is a valuable addition to the therapeutic program. Most programs use cognitive-behavioral therapy or a DBT-based therapeutic approach. Although of high importance, parent management training and other evidence-based practices such as motivational interviewing (MI) and interpersonal psychotherapy (IPT) are not suited for therapeutic milieus. These other treatment options are longer term than most hospital stays and more suitable for an outpatient setting rather than a crisis stabilization setting such as an inpatient unit. **(p. 1024)**

Reference

Trask EV, Fawley-King K, Garland AF, et al: Do aftercare services reduce risk of psychiatric rehospitalization for children? Psychol Serv 13(2):127–132, 2016 26147361

C H A P T E R   4 7

School-Based Interventions

Erika Ryst, M.D.

Jeff Q. Bostic, M.D., Ed.D.

Sharon A. Hoover, Ph.D.

Kris Scardamalia, Ph.D., LSSP, LP

1. All of the following are components of a comprehensive school mental health program *except*

A. Psychiatric medication management services delivered in the school setting.
B. Collaboration between school and community partners.
C. Mental health screening, early identification of problems, and triage to appropriate levels of support.
D. Multitiered evidence-based interventions to promote mental health.

The correct response is Option A: Psychiatric medication management services delivered in the school setting.

National best practice standards now call for a model of comprehensive school mental health, which involves 1) collaboration between school and community partners to offer a full continuum of mental health supports and services in schools; 2) mental health screening and monitoring to identify concerns early and triage students for appropriate levels of support; and 3) multitiered, evidence-based interventions to promote mental health for all students (tier 1), to support students with emerging or mild mental health symptoms (tier 2), and to treat students with mental illness (tier 3). Although medication management is a tier 3 intervention that a child psychiatrist may recommend, a comprehensive school mental health program can provide these services either directly within a school or by collaborating with a community provider or organization outside the school setting. **(pp. 1045, 1047)**

2. Which of the following is true regarding a Section 504 plan that is generated by a school for a student?

    A. It enables the student to receive classroom accommodations by regular education staff.
    B. It provides specialized instruction for the student.
    C. It modifies the curriculum by lowering academic standards.
    D. It provides the same legal protections as an individualized education program (IEP).

    The correct response is Option A: It enables the student to receive classroom accommodations by regular education staff.

    As part of a 504 plan, students may be identified with a disability but not require specialized instruction or a change in the educational setting. Classroom accommodations by regular education staff may be sufficient for these students to make educational progress. These plans derive from Section 504 of the Rehabilitation Act (Office for Civil Rights 2010), which ensures that all disabled children receive a "free and appropriate public education" in the "least restrictive environment." *Accommodations* refer to classroom changes that help students meet requirements without "lowering" academic standards. Parents may also request a school evaluation to determine if a disability is present and interferes with their child's educational progress. The request is usually provided in writing to the school's principal or student support team leader. A 504 plan does not provide the same requirements or protections (e.g., annual review meetings, reevaluations every 3 years) as for students who qualify for special education. **(p. 1048)**

3. A child psychiatrist is a consultant for her local school district and also provides direct services to students within the school. One of her direct service patients is not receiving needed speech therapy services that are listed on the patient's IEP. What should the child psychiatrist do when addressing this issue?

    A. Clarify that her primary role for this case is as the child's provider.
    B. Respect the fact that it is up to the school's discretion to follow her suggestions.
    C. Work with administrative staff to develop quality control procedures that ensure that all IEPs are implemented correctly.
    D. Leave it to the child's pediatrician to advocate for the child's school services in order to avoid a conflict of interest.

    The correct response is Option A: Clarify that her primary role for this case is as the child's provider.

    If the child psychiatrist functions both as a consultant and as a direct provider for students in the school, these two roles may conflict. The child psychiatrist should always clarify the primary role for that case (consultant or provider) before engaging with a school to address a specific mental health issue or student.

The other options reflect the potential actions of a child psychiatrist who functions as a consultant. The child psychiatrist who functions as a consultant recognizes that 1) the child psychiatrist is providing suggestions to the school (usually the school staff), but the decisions in response to these suggestions are at the school's discretion alone, and the school may follow all, parts, or none of the psychiatrist's suggestions; 2) any suggestions should be designed to benefit most of the students at the school and not only the identified student; 3) the psychiatrist does not have a doctor-patient relationship with the student. Advocacy for a specific student to attain certain services or placement should be done by the clinician who is providing direct treatment. **(p. 1052)**

4. Which of the following best describes the role of a school psychologist?

    A. The majority of their time is spent conducting psychological assessments.
    B. They are the primary providers of psychosocial interventions in schools.
    C. They assist students in college or vocational planning and academic planning.
    D. They act as a liaison between the school and the community.

    The correct response is Option A: The majority of their time is spent conducting psychological assessments.

    School psychologists either are employed by the school or have a contract with the school. School psychologists are trained in consultation, psychoeducational assessment, and counseling strategies. Given current workforce shortages, the majority of their time is often focused on conducting and interpreting psychological assessments to determine eligibility for special education services and assisting in developing IEPs.

    School adjustment counselors and social workers provide psychosocial interventions to students and sometimes to their families.

    School counselors (formerly referred to as guidance counselors) sometimes provide psychotherapy to students, although in secondary schools they often primarily assist students in college or vocational planning and academic planning, including class selection.

    School administrators act as a liaison between the school and the community. **(pp. 1053–1054)**

5. Bounce Back is a targeted small-group school-based intervention for at-risk students with symptoms of which of the following?

    A. Trauma.
    B. Anxiety.
    C. Depression.
    D. Substance misuse.

The correct response is Option A: Trauma.

Bounce Back (http://bouncebackprogram.org) is a group-based CBT trauma-focused treatment for kindergarten through fifth-grade children.

Coping Cat is a 16-session CBT intervention for students ages 7–13 years with anxiety (Podell et al. 2010).

Adolescent Coping with Depression (CWD-A; www.saavsus.com/adolescent-coping-with-depression-course) is a group therapy to address symptoms of depression in adolescents.

Strengthening Families Program (SFP; https://strengtheningfamiliesprogram.org) is a skills training youth and parent program that teaches parenting skills and youth life and refusal skills. **(pp. 1059–1061, Table 47–3)**

6.   A psychiatrist is asked to consult on a fifth-grade student with a learning disorder and ADHD. The teacher reports that the student repeatedly gets out of his seat and distracts the class with jokes when the class is asked to read independently and silently. The teacher is frustrated because she has redirected the student from this behavior numerous times without effect. She says, "I just want to find some strategies that will get him to stop disrupting the class." Which of the following consultation tactics would be most useful for the psychiatrist to employ at this time?

A. Suggest that the student may be using these behaviors to distract from the fact that he struggles with reading.
B. Praise the teacher for her perseverance in repeatedly redirecting the student.
C. Backtrack to the teacher's original intention to improve the students' reading skills.
D. Use the teacher's own words, "strategies that will get him to stop disrupting the class," to frame the intervention.

The correct response is Option A: Suggest that the student may be using these behaviors to distract from the fact that he struggles with reading.

Maladaptive student behaviors may be used to solve problems when no other solution is available. By helping the teacher see the child differently, the child psychiatrist consultant opens the teacher up to consider other intervention strategies. In this case, the student may need more individual attention or help during independent reading tasks.

Although it is helpful to praise school staff for their creative and effective efforts, in this case, the teacher's perseverance caused her to continue an ineffective practice, so it would not be helpful to praise her for this specific behavior.

When students or staff act inappropriately, the consultant can refer to the good intention that motivated the person's (mis)behavior so that self-esteem, and thus willingness to attempt different behaviors, is maximized. Appealing to the teacher's intrinsic and altruistic motives might be appropriate, but in this situation, it would be less helpful than getting the teacher to see the student differently.

Similarly, although framing interventions with terms used by staff can increase the person's feeling of being heard and improves the probability that they will invest in proposed solutions, in this case, the most effective approach is to help the teacher realize that the student's behavior stems from his difficulty with reading. These two strategies could possibly be combined by using such language as "providing him with individual help during reading time may be a strategy that will get him to stop disrupting the class." **(pp. 1054–1056)**

7. According to the University of Virginia's Comprehensive School Threat Assessment Guidelines, which of the following indicates that the school can likely screen out a threat as transient?

   A. When the threat is an expression of humor, anger, or frustration.
   B. When the threat includes a detailed plan to harm.
   C. When the threat involves peers in the planning.
   D. When the threat includes proclamations such as "something big will happen next week."

   The correct response is Option A: When the threat is an expression of humor, anger, or frustration.

   According to the University of Virginia's Comprehensive School Threat Assessment Guidelines (available at www.curry.virginia.edu/youth-violence-project), an evaluator can attempt to resolve the threat as transient when it is an expression of humor, anger, or frustration; when there is no intent to harm; and when the student is able to retract, explain, or apologize to indicate they have no future intent to harm anyone.
   Threats are more serious if they 1) include plausible details (e.g., plans, methods, people); 2) have been discussed with multiple people over an identifiable period of time; 3) show evidence of a plan (and planning); 4) involve peers in the planning or enactment of the threat; 5) include proclamations or awareness of others about the threat event (e.g., "something big will happen at this time"); and 6) are consistent with physical evidence such as weaponry obtained or information showing efforts to build weapons or traps. **(p. 1063)**

References

Office for Civil Rights: Free Appropriate Public Education for Students With Disabilities: Requirements Under Section 504 of the Rehabilitation Act of 1973.Washington, DC, U.S. Department of Education, August 2010. Available at: www2.ed.gov/about/offices/list/ocr/docs/edlite-FAPE504.html. Accessed October 29, 2020.
Podell JL, Mychailyszyn M, Edmunds J, et al: The Coping Cat Program for anxious youth: the FEAR plan comes to life. Cogn Behav Pract 17(2):132–141, 2010

CHAPTER 48

Collaborating
With Primary Care

Elise Fallucco, M.D.

Rachel Ballard, M.D., M.A.

1.   Which of the following is the largest benefit of integrated or collaborative care models compared with traditional outpatient care?

A. Integrated or collaborative care models enable child and adolescent psychiatrists (CAPs) to provide long-term care for patients in pediatric settings.
B. Reimbursement is higher for clinical services in an integrated or collaborative care model.
C. Integrated or collaborative care models facilitate treatment for a larger population of youth.
D. Patients with severe, complex psychopathology can be managed in a pediatric setting using integrated or collaborative care models.

The correct response is Option C: Integrated or collaborative care models facilitate treatment for a larger population of youth.

By partnering with pediatricians, CAPs who practice integrated or collaborative care have increased capacity to care for a much larger caseload than do CAPs who practice traditional outpatient care. In traditional outpatient care, CAPs provide long-term care for patients with severe, complex psychopathology, limiting their ability to see new patients. Because of challenges with reimbursement for clinical services, most entities that use integrated or collaborative care models need to receive state or philanthropic funding. **(p. 1072)**

2. Who serves as the director of the care team in the University of Washington AIMS Center model of collaborative care?

A. The child and adolescent psychiatrist.
B. The primary care provider.
C. The behavioral health care coordinator.
D. The parent(s) or caregiver(s) of the child.

The correct response is Option B: The primary care provider.

The AIMS Center model of collaborative care places the primary care provider as the director of the care team who is responsible for identifying and treating patients. The behavioral health care coordinator and the consulting child and adolescent psychiatrist support the primary care provider. Although the parents or caregivers of the child are involved in family-centered care, they do not direct the care team. **(pp. 1073–1074)**

3. Which of the following distinguishes the consultative collaboration model from child psychiatry access programs?

A. The consultative collaboration model allows psychiatrists to care for a larger population than is typically served by child psychiatry access programs.
B. The consultative collaboration model is often supported by state-level funding.
C. The consultative collaboration model provides primarily same-day telephone consultation.
D. The consultative collaboration model allows psychiatrists to personally examine patients and provide a higher level of consultation.

The correct response is Option D: The consultative collaboration model allows psychiatrists to personally examine patients and provide a higher level of consultation.

Child psychiatry access programs provide primarily same-day telephone consultation for pediatric clinicians. They are typically supported by state-level funding and serve a much larger population than can be served using the consultative collaboration model. The consultative collaboration model delivers outpatient consultation, allowing psychiatrists to examine patients and provide a higher level of consultation to the referring pediatric clinician. **(pp. 1073–1074)**

4. Which of the following strategies can facilitate primary care clinician engagement in collaborative care models?

A. Identify champions within the pediatric practice.
B. Implement training in a convenient and accessible format for clinicians.
C. Develop a plan for ongoing consultation.
D. All of the above.

The correct response is Option D: All of the above.

The strategies for facilitating primary care clinician engagement in collaborative care models include identifying champions within the pediatric practice, implementing training in a convenient and accessible format for clinicians, and developing a plan for ongoing consultation. **(p. 1079)**

5. In models of collaborative care in which a mental health clinician has not directly evaluated the patient, what is the most appropriate way to give recommendations?

    A. "In cases like these, we generally titrate the antidepressant if there has been minimal improvement after 4 weeks."
    B. "For this patient, I would increase the sertraline from 50 mg to 100 mg."
    C. "Switch from sertraline to fluoxetine if there is no response."
    D. "For this patient, I would recommend genetic testing."

    The correct response is Option A: "In cases like these, we generally titrate the antidepressant if there has been minimal improvement after 4 weeks."

    The consulting psychiatrist should communicate their recommendation using a general statement such as "In cases such as the one you are describing, it is usually helpful to start a low-dose antidepressant medication and refer for cognitive-behavioral therapy." This wording clarifies that the consulting psychiatrist provides general advice and education regarding mental health care rather than specific medical advice for a patient. **(p. 1080)**

6. Which of the following is true regarding the financing of collaborative care models?

    A. Collaborative care codes currently approved by the Centers for Medicare and Medicaid Services allow psychiatrists to bill for time spent in collaborative care activities.
    B. There is no evidence that collaborative care for adolescent depression is cost-effective in clinical systems.
    C. Consulting psychiatrists who see patients face-to-face for evaluation and treatment planning in collaboration with the primary care pediatrician can bill standard evaluation and management plans for these visits.
    D. Value-based payment systems are financially incompatible with most collaborative models.

    The correct response is Option C: Consulting psychiatrists who see patients face-to-face for evaluation and treatment planning in collaboration with the primary care pediatrician can bill standard evaluation and management plans for these visits.

As currently approved by the Centers for Medicare and Medicaid Services, the collaborative care codes allow primary care clinicians, but not psychiatrists, to bill. Initial studies have shown that collaborative care for adolescent depression is cost-effective for the system as a whole. Value-based payment systems may incentivize collaborative care. Similar to traditional outpatient care, face-to-face evaluation and treatment of patients can be reimbursed using standard evaluation and management codes. **(pp. 1080–1081)**

CHAPTER 49

Collaborating With Inpatient and Subspecialty Pediatrics

Jill Weissberg-Benchell, Ph.D.

1. William is a 16-year-old recently diagnosed with non-Hodgkin's lymphoma. He is actively working with his teachers to modify his homework assignments to accommodate the demands of his chemotherapy. This style of coping is known as which of the following?

    A. Secondary control coping.
    B. Emotional expression coping.
    C. Primary control coping.
    D. Behavioral activation coping.

    The correct response is Option C: Primary control coping.

    Coping responses focused on efforts to directly change a source of stress (homework is a source of stress; problem-solving is the coping response) is called *primary control coping*.
        Other coping responses are focused on adapting to the stress through cognitive-behavioral techniques such as reappraisal, positive thinking, distraction, and acceptance. This approach is often called secondary control coping. Emotional expression and behavioral activation are not examples of coping styles. **(p. 1088)**

2. Resilience influences how individuals adapt to a chronic illness and includes which of the following constructs?

    A. Understanding the purpose behind the daily demands of the treatment regimen.
    B. Building skills necessary to promote psychosocial well-being.

C. Being in the action stage in the stages of change model.

D. Developing adaptive emotion regulation skills.

The correct response is Option B: Building skills necessary to promote psychosocial well-being.

Most families tend to be resilient and cope well with chronic illness. Hilliard et al. (2012) defined resilience as being able to achieve one or more positive outcomes despite exposure to significant risk or adversity. The collaborating behavioral health specialist's goals should include helping families develop the tools and skills necessary to promote psychosocial well-being, high quality of life, and resilience to help them overcome the challenges of chronic illness. The other options do not pertain to the concept of resilience. **(p. 1088)**

3.   The consultant and pediatric clinicians are in the same space within the same facility as a team with shared systems and communicate regularly in which of the following models of pediatric consultation-liaison (CL) psychiatry?

A. Coordinated care model.

B. Co-located care model.

C. Integrated care model.

D. Proactive psychiatric consultation programs model.

The correct response is Option C: Integrated care model.

Coordinated care refers to a model in which the consultant and the pediatric team are in separate facilities or systems and communicate intermittently as requested by the pediatric team.

In *co-located care*, the consultant and the pediatric team are in the same facility with some shared systems and frequently communicate about shared patients.

In the *integrated care* model, the consultant and pediatric clinicians are in the same space within the same facility as a team with shared systems and communicate regularly.

Co-located and integrated care models are thought to be the most effective for outpatient specialty services or inpatient medical settings.

Proactive psychiatric consultation programs are a new model of providing rapid inpatient mental health consultations to adult patients admitted to a medical service with current medical and behavioral health needs that have the potential to interfere with the delivery of care. This is a developing concept in pediatric CL psychiatry, and only a few programs exist nationwide. **(p. 1085)**

4.   All of the following medications are *not* tightly protein bound except

A. Sertraline.

B. Lithium.

C. Methylphenidate.

D. Venlafaxine.

The correct response is Option A: Sertraline.

Pharmacokinetics involves the absorption, distribution, and metabolism of medications. Medical illness that affects certain organ systems can alter pharmacokinetics. Most psychotropic medications are tightly protein bound. Exceptions are lithium, venlafaxine, divalproex sodium, methylphenidate, gabapentin, and topiramate. Sertraline and other selective serotonin reuptake inhibitors (SSRIs) are tightly protein bound. **(p. 1092)**

5. Which of the following is true regarding the use of psychiatric medications in patients with comorbid epilepsy?

   A. Psychotropic medications are usually not a concern in epilepsy patients because they increase the seizure threshold.
   B. SSRIs, trazodone, and the α-agonists are particularly unsafe to use in patients with comorbid psychiatric illness and epilepsy.
   C. Lithium is considered an anticonvulsant and can always be used safely in epilepsy patients.
   D. Substantial data suggest that stimulants can be used safely, particularly when seizures are well controlled.

The correct response is Option D: Substantial data suggest that stimulants can be used safely, particularly when seizures are well controlled.

Psychotropic medications should be used with caution in patients with epilepsy, primarily because many of these medications lower the seizure threshold.

SSRIs, trazodone, and the α-agonists are safe to use in patients with comorbid psychiatric illness and epilepsy.

Lithium is considered a proconvulsant but can be used with care in appropriate cases.

The FDA medication guides for stimulants (www.fda.gov) list seizures as serious side effects, especially in patients with an underlying history of seizures, and the *Physicians' Desk Reference* warns about the risk of methylphenidate lowering the seizure threshold. However, substantial data suggest that stimulants can be used safely, particularly when seizures are well controlled. No evidence indicates that long-term use of stimulants increases the risk for seizures. **(p. 1096)**

Reference

Hilliard ME, Harris MA, Weissberg-Benchell J: Diabetes resilience: a model of risk and protection in type 1 diabetes. Curr Diab Rep 12(6):739–748, 2012 22956459